Pathways in Medical Ethics

Alan G Johnson,
M.A., M.Chir., F.R.C.S.

Professor of Surgery, University of Sheffield

Edward Arnold
A division of Hodder & Stoughton
LONDON   MELBOURNE   AUCKLAND

© 1990 Alan G. Johnson

First published in Great Britain 1990

British Library Cataloguing in Publication Data

Johnson A. G. (Alan Godfrey)
  Pathways in medical ethics.
  1. Medicine. Ethical aspects
  I. Title
  174′.2

  ISBN 0–340–50720–9

Whilst the advice and information in this book is believed to be true and accurate at the date of going to press, neither the author nor the publisher can accept any legal responsibility or liability for any errors or omissions that may be made. In particular (but without limiting the generality of the preceding disclaimer) every effort has been made to check drug dosages; however, it is still possible that errors have been missed. Furthermore, dosage schedules are being continually revised and new side-effects recognized. For these reasons the reader is strongly urged to consult the drug companies' printed instructions before administering any of the drugs recommended in this book.

Typeset in 10/11 Palatino by Anneset, Weston-super-Mare, Avon
Printed and bound in Great Britain for Edward Arnold, a division of Hodder and Stoughton Limited, Mill Road, Dunton Green, Sevenoaks, Kent TN13 2YA by Richard Clay Ltd, Bungay, Suffolk.

Contents

Preface

To the many medical students with whom
I have discussed these matters over the years

Sapere Aude – Dare to be wise
Horace

The modern doctor cannot escape ethical issues and newly qualified House Officers often feel ill prepared to face these moral dilemmas. Although some are debated by the media and discussed in formal and informal student groups, there is little guidance about the basis and method of ethical decision-making. Often the student's best hope is for a convenient 'rule of thumb', or for inspiration to arrive at the time of crisis.

This book aims to provide guidance through the ethical maze and to show that ethical decisions can follow a logical, rather than an arbitrary process – that there is no need to rely on inspired guesswork or secondhand advice. It is felt that the concept of pathways (or algorithms) is helpful, as students are used to thinking in this way when analysing pathways of surgical or medical management for their patients. Pathways, like ethical thinking, can diverge from a common starting point or converge to the same destination from very different starting points or moral bases. There are many branches and decisions on the way and not a few blind alleys! Some pathways, like some clinical problems, are relatively straightforward, while others are devious and tortuous.

Within this framework, the overall aim has been to provide a relatively simple book which will emphasise the four principles required in the teaching of ethics to students in the health sciences:

1. Awareness of ethical problems.
2. Discussion of the moral basis for ethical decisions.
3. Methods of analysing and thinking about ethical problems.
4. Awareness of existing guidelines, legal judgements and ethical committees.

Although primarily written for medical students, most of the text will be useful to many members of the caring professions, especially as, nowadays, ethical problems are commonly discussed in multidisciplinary groups. Clinical examples are given, including the common, less dramatic problems, which are often forgotten by the media; but the aim is not to give 'maps' for all possible clinical situations nor to go over all the well-worn arguments again, but to equip the readers to find the paths for themselves.

The chapters cover the syllabus that all medical students should be expected to know and understand, when they study ethics as part of the medical curriculum. A number will wish to delve into the subject more deeply and read more widely. The suggestions for

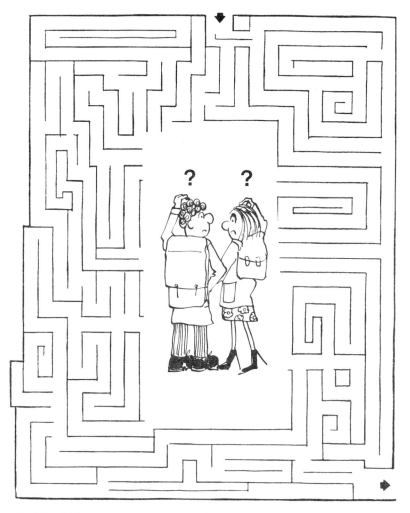

The Ethical Maze

further reading are not intended to be exhaustive but are selected to give an entry into the very extensive literature. Some universities and institutes are now providing courses leading to diplomas or degrees and they will have their own more detailed syllabuses and reading lists. It is hoped that the format will show that ethics is as interesting and as relevant to clinical practice as any other part of medical training.

Sheffield, 1990   Alan G Johnson

Acknowledgements

I am very grateful to Mr David R Millar FRCS (Ed) FRCOG and to Dr Paul Johnson MB ChB for helpful suggestions during the preparation of this book, and to my wife Esther for her continual support and help with checking and proof-reading. I am indebted to Mr Pat Elliot for the drawings and Mrs Josie Wilson for typing the manuscript.

Part 1
Finding the paths

1 Definitions

'Why study such a boring subject as medical ethics?'
'Medical ethics is for professors of philosophy in ivory towers!'
'There are no solutions, so why bother to discuss it?'
'Most of the issues do not concern us, as students'
'Once you have done euthanasia, abortion and embryo research,
there is not much more to discuss'

These are some of the adverse reactions to a textbook or course on medical ethics. The answer is that you have no option but to study medical ethics! You cannot escape them, because they are an integral part of medical practice and unless you think about them beforehand, you will suddenly find yourself having to make an urgent ethical decision completely unprepared. Unfortunately, the study of ethics is not a hobby, like golf, playing the guitar or knitting, which you can take up if and when you wish. It is not even a branch of medicine you can choose to specialize in, such as pathology or paediatrics. All branches of health care have ethical involvement.

In Britain, we have paid lip-service to the teaching of medical ethics in our medical schools for years, but often it has amounted to no more than the occasional formal lecture or discussion after a ward round. It was felt that ethics were assimilated by diffusion from the example of 'our chiefs'. That these gentlemen were not always paragons of virtue was conveniently overlooked. An example — valuable as it may be — must be reinforced by more formal teaching. The working party on the Teaching of Medical Ethics, under the chairmanship of the late Sir Desmond Pond, reported in 1987, and it considered the principles and the methods of teaching. The report encourages diversity and recommends that the teaching should permeate all parts of the course and should remain relevant to practical clinical problems. Small group seminars are particularly recommended rather than formal, didactic lectures.

We cannot consider medical ethics in isolation. In fact, it could be argued that they do not exist at all. Medicine, like any other scientific enterprise, cannot produce ethical principles; it can only raise ethical problems and be a forum in which ethical principles can be put into practice. Medical ethics only develop when doctors and other health workers bring their personal or corporate ethical systems and apply them to the medical field, in just the same way politicians and nuclear scientists may bring their ethical principles to their own spheres of influence. We must not therefore discuss medical ethics as if they were divorced from the ethics of everyday life. They are special only because they often deal with issues of life and death, and there is usually an urgency about the decisions. But in the political and military arenas, decisions may affect the life and death of thousands of people; and even in everyday civilian life, a bus driver travelling down a slippery road who sees a child run in front of the bus has to make a split-second decision whether to brake suddenly and try to save one life but risk the lives of 50 passengers, or continue moving and sacrifice one life to protect his passengers.

It will, therefore, help our thinking throughout this book if we see medical ethics as just one special branch of general ethics. For example, the question about telling the truth to patients is only a particular example of the principle of telling the truth in the family, the business-world and in everyday life. Despite this, however, a body of opinion becomes accepted by a profession and becomes known as 'it's ethics'.

Definition

Professor Dunstan (qv) has given an excellent definition of medical ethics:

> the obligations of a moral nature which govern the practice of medicine

There are three key words in that definition:

Obligations   Ethics are not merely an excuse for a good debate. There are obligations involved — things we ought and ought not to do. One cannot discuss medical ethics as if one was expressing a view on clothes fashions or different hairstyles. One part of medical ethics is descriptive, but because something happens it does not mean that it is right in medicine or in other walks of life. It is easy to assume that the norm is necessarily right and familiarity with a course of action may numb the critical faculty. This occurs particularly when we have to take a decision that is the 'lesser of two evils'. After a very short time we forget that it was an evil and assume it is right and good.

The concept of rights and duties within ethics is classified as 'deontological' theory, as opposed to 'teleological' theory which is based on effects and consequences. Deontological theory is often associated with ethics that have a religious basis and teleological ethics are championed by utilitarianists. The former may be summarized as 'doing the right thing' and the latter as 'doing the thing right'. We will return to these later, but most doctors probably include both aspects in their decision-making: the obligations are tempered by the likely consequences of an action and the results are checked against duties and obligations.

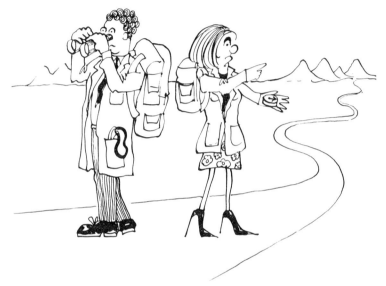

Figure 1.1 The teleologist tries to see where decisions lead. The deontologist (on the right) travels in a planned direction.

'Moral' The words 'moral' and 'ethical' are often interchangeable and unfortunately the word 'ethical' gives the impression of academics at ancient universities, set apart from the real world. 'Moral dilemmas' in medicine or the 'morality of decisions' make it all sound more realistic and down-to-earth.

Morals are concerned with right and wrong and with good and bad. In practice, it is not always so clear-cut and we are often concerned with what is better or worse. It is not the moral principles in themselves that are unclear but, when applied, they may conflict with other principles, as we shall see in the course of this book.

Morals must have a basis; they do not 'just happen' and different religious and or philosophical bases will lead to very different courses of action.

An analysis of ethical systems is of some interest but does not lead to a reason for a moral stance. As Thompson (1987) points out, the basic principles of medical ethics cannot be assumed to be self-evident just because they are embalmed in traditional medical practice. Their claims need to be justified from outside medicine. The various bases will be discussed in Chapter 5, but it is becoming increasingly difficult to establish an agreed ethical position in most societies today, when there is such a wide variation in the moral bases. It is important to stress, at this point, that those who say they have no religion and no philosophy of right and wrong, are also taking a moral position which will affect their practice of medicine. A 'negative' position is just as much a stance as a 'positive' one.

Govern It is germane to this definition of medical ethics that the morals govern the medical practice rather than vice versa. The medical dilemma does not provide the morals. Morals have to be brought to bear on a particular dilemma. What *does* happen cannot automatically become what *should* happen. Sadly, in the history of medical advances this has often occurred. Usually the philosophers and ethicists are well behind the advances in science and are running to catch up, rather than controlling the pace. The Warnock Committee, which was a response to research in reproductive medicine that had already started, has tried to plan ahead and control the direction of this research in Britain.

The term 'situational ethics' has come to imply that the situation will provide the poor confused doctor with the answer at the time, from his experience and his knowledge of the likely outcome. Situational ethics can also mean that moral principles are applied to a particular situation and decisions cannot be made in the abstract. This distinction brings us to one of the classical debates in philosophy. Whilst Kant taught that principles must be established before their application to a situation, the existentialists, such as Sartre, believed the truth and validity lie only in the individual's experience and not apart from this. For Sartre, ethical principles could not be deduced from basic premises about the world and then applied to a clinical situation. For him there is no external obligation; any 'ought' is entirely self-imposed.

The details and implications of the different world views will be discussed in more detail in later sections.

An agreed ethic?

Given the many different bases and approaches to ethics, particularly in a multicultural society like modern Britain, it seems increasingly difficult to obtain agreement within professions such as medicine and other healthcare groups. Many hope that from a discussion between people of different views, a general consensus will arise. What usually comes from such an approach is the lowest common denominator of all views, which amounts to very little. A cook, who fills and stirs a dish with a variety of unplanned and unweighed ingredients produces an indefinable mush; whereas an experienced cook follows a well-tried recipe. In ethics, it is more profitable to analyse and define the different world views and to follow the consequences of applying them in medicine. That is why this book follows a theme of pathways and at the present time these pathways are diverging rather than converging. However, there is a general conservatism within well-established professions that discourages its members from putting their own philosophies into practice rather than adopting the majority view. For example, it is unusual to see an evolutionary humanist pushing his philosophy, of the survival of the fittest and the physical improvement of the human race, to its logical conclusion within medicine. Hitler started to do so but largely in a political rather than a medical framework.

Despite many different opinions, there *has* been agreement, embodied in codes or conventions in a number of areas of medical activity, such as organ transplantation and research patients. They will be referred to in Chapter 12, but by their very nature they can only be guidelines rather than detailed instructions.

The scope of medical ethics

From the foregoing introduction, it is clear that medical ethics have a number of facets. These will be explored later in this book, but are summarized here.

Awareness

It is the job of ethical teaching to call attention to the implications of our actions, both personal and professional. Many health workers, especially during training, are unaware of some of the more mundane ethical issues, such as confidentiality, although they are very conscious of those issues commonly debated in the media, such as abortion or euthanasia. Indeed, it is very easy for junior nurses or medical secretaries to break the patients' confidences without even realizing it, merely by answering an apparently innocent enquiry on the telephone. So it is important to encourage debate and raise questions — but raising them does not necessarily solve them! How many hours must have been spent in fruitless debate because there was no framework for the discussion!

Analysis

The study of analytical or philosophical ethics is concerned with how decisions are made and the principles on which they are made. This is important in order to provide the framework for careful ethical thinking, and a considerable part of this book will be dedicated to the analysis of problems. It is very easy to assume that two actions are very similar, when, on further analysis, the ethical issues are quite distinct. For example, much of the confusion in the euthanasia debate has been due to the failure to define terms. Switching off the respirator when a patient has been declared brain dead has sometimes been equated with the giving of a lethal injection to a fully alert patient with an incurable disease. As we shall see, many everyday actions have very little, if any, ethical content and it is easy for an ethical enthusiast to see dilemmas around every corner or under every hospital bed! Philosophical ethics must also ask how the principles that govern a particular doctor's action are derived.

Codes and declarations

It is entirely proper that ethical codes, declarations or conventions should be drawn up to act as guidelines, but they are only valuable if they are used as intended and not as a substitute for the individual's own conscience. It is easy to shelter behind a code to avoid thinking through the real issues.

Bases

As we have already seen, a moral system must have a basis, so in ethical discussion we must continually ask the question 'why?' 'Why are human beings valuable?' 'On what moral basis should you tell the truth?' Most of the people coming into our healthcare professions have not asked themselves these questions but have adopted the views of their peers or parents and assumed they are right. There may, of course, be several different moral bases for the same course of action. The Hindu, the Christian and the Humanist may all agree it is wrong to kill another innocent human being, but for different reasons. In the same way, they may agree that inflicting suffering on animals was also wrong: the Hindu, because he believes in reincarnation and that the animal might possess the soul of one of his relations, the Christian because he believes that he is responsible to God for the way he treats other parts of God's creation, and the Humanist because cruelty to another animal demeans the pre-eminent standing of the human animal. It is a business of ethics to explore and define these reasons.

The place of conscience

The human conscience is an indicator and has to be informed and educated. It is possible to train one's conscience in such a way that it will respond to good as if it were evil — and vice versa — or just to suppress its function altogether. However, many would argue, from varying religious traditions, that there is some intrinsic sense of right and wrong, of fairness and justice, within each of us that will break through even a most oppressive attempt to subdue it. However, an appeal to a kind of infallible 'inner intuition' is likely to be unrewarding on the spur of the moment. Even the Christian's dependence on the prayer and guidance in a crisis is no substitute for careful thinking and planning beforehand, whenever this is possible. It is our responsibility to keep our consciences as alert and informed as possible.

The place of a profession

Traditionally, the essence of a profession is that it is responsible for setting and maintaining its own standards and for disciplining its own members for breaches of those standards. It is, therefore, right that a profession should develop as consistent a body of opinion as possible; but modern medical advances are so complex, and the profession so involved in them, that it is important to have responsible people from other fields to advise on ethical matters. This principle has been embodied in the setting up of Hospital Ethical Committees in Britain and the Institutional Review Committees in the United States.

On the other hand, there is a danger that the profession will abdicate its responsibility. Some voices are heard to say 'We are servants of society and it is up to society to work out what it wants us to do, and we will do it.' This could lead to a dangerous control of a profession's ethics by a totalitarian government, a situation which has arisen in the last fifty years in more than one country. The role of the doctor in relation to the state laws with which he disagrees will be discussed later (p. 66).

Etiquette

Etiquette is a pattern of behaviour within a certain group in society, e.g. a profession. It is concerned with good relationships between the members, but is not usually concerned with major moral issues. For example, it is good etiquette for the consultant to reply promptly to a general practitioner's letter of referral. This does not usually affect the care of the patient immediately (although it might if the patient's drug regimen had been changed and the general practitioner was unaware of this). It is good etiquette for a consultant physician, whose opinion has been asked for by a surgeon, to discuss the problem with that surgeon before referring the patient to a specialist colleague. This is unlikely to affect the patient's treatment, but jealousies and poor relationships between hospital staff are detrimental to the patient in the end. The same principles apply to general practice and to the branches of the nursing profession.

Until recently, etiquette and ethics were often confused even in official publications, but they are now becoming more clearly understood.

Expectations — false and true

Like the alchemists of old, who were always searching for the magic stone that would turn all to gold, the modern student lives in constant hope that there is a magic formula that will take the thinking and emotional tension out of ethical decisions. This is a false expectation, for life is not like that! We can clarify the issues, outline the decision-making process, explore the principles and supply guidelines, but it is never easy and it is likely to become more difficult in the future.

Many students feel there is something wrong with *them* if they find it difficult to resolve these conflicts. Dilemmas are always difficult to resolve and decisions involving people will always have some emotional aspects (unless the doctor has become so hardened that he or she is concerned no longer). So if you find these problems difficult, take heart; you are in good company and it shows you still have the concern for people and awareness of the problems that produce the tension!

However, the solution of ethical problems is becoming more and more urgent as technology accelerates rapidly. It is not enough to discuss endlessly while the scientific world moves on. Solutions are urgently needed and this is a *right* expectation of medical ethics. The problem lies in those who study ethics, both inside and outside the medical profession, who are afraid of being unpopular and of being accused of 'halting progress'. But those who are concerned about human values must not be afraid to suggest limits and controls to research; that is their responsibility. Otherwise we return to science dictating morality with an authority it does not possess.

References and Further Reading

Dunstan GR (1974). *The Artifice of Ethics* SCM Press, London.

Dunstan GR (1981). In *Dictionary of Medical Ethics* (Ed) Duncan AS, Dunstan GR and Welbourn RB. Darton Longman and Todd, London.

Gillon R (1986). *Philosophical Medical Ethics* John Wiley, Chichester.

Johnson AG (1983). Teaching medical ethics as a practical subject: observations from experience. *Journal of Medical Ethics*; **9**: 5–7.

Jonsen AR, Siegler M and Winslade WJ (1982). *Clinical Ethics*. McMillan, London, New York, Toronto.

Lacey AR (1979). *A Dictionary of Philosophy*. Routledge and Kegan Paul, London.

Lockwood M (1986). *Moral Dilemmas in Modern Medicine*. Oxford University Press, Oxford.

Thompson IE (1987). Fundamental ethical principles, in health care. *British Medical Journal*; **295**: 1461–5.

Working Party on the teaching of medical ethics (1987). (Chairman) Sir Desmond Pond. Institute of Medical Ethics, London.

2 Pathways in the past: historical perspectives

Every schoolboy knows that doctors take the Hippocratic Oath on qualification and practice by its precepts unswervingly for the rest of their lives. Every schoolboy is wrong! Few doctors have taken the Hippocratic Oath in Britain for many years, although this used to happen, especially in the older universities. Most medical students and doctors have only a vague idea about what the Oath contains and, if they knew that they would be asked to 'Swear by Apollo the Physician, and Asclepius and Hygieia and Panacea, and all the gods and goddesses' they might regard it less seriously! However, at least one medical school has recently introduced a statement of ethical principles which graduands of the medical faculty are reminded about at their degree ceremony (see Appendix I).

Medical ethics are not new, and writings about the duties and responsibilities of doctors and healers go back to antiquity, even earlier than the Greeks. The history of medical ethics can be divided into four periods:

1. Ancient times
2. The Middle Ages
3. 1600–1900 — the modern period
4. 1940 to the present day

We will have a brief look at the important contributions from different sources, but examine the Hippocratic Oath and the recent declarations in more detail.

Ancient times

Ancient Hebrew writings

In a number of places in the Talmud there are passages about the high moral standards and responsibilities expected of physicians.

HISTORICAL PATHWAYS — I

ANCIENT TIMES:

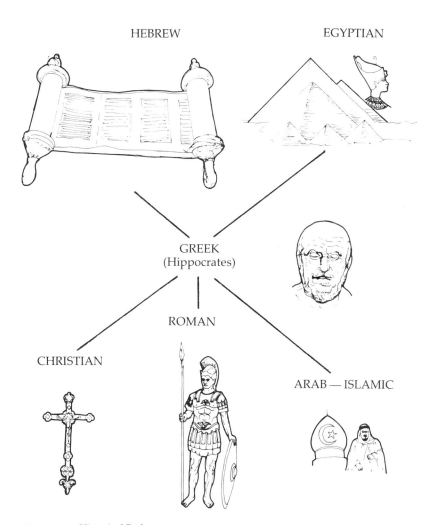

Figure 2.1 Historical Pathways

There are instructions about the fees and about the ethical dilemmas of obstetrics. Permission is given for Caesarean section to save the child if a mother has died in labour, but feticide is allowed if it is necessary to save the mother:

> Should a woman have a difficult delivery, the child is cut up in her womb and taken out limb by limb, for her life comes first. However, if most of the child has come out, it may not be harmed — for one life should not be sacrificed for another
>
> *Ohalot* **7**: 6

Ancient Egyptian writings

Sophisticated medicine existed in ancient Egypt and is described in the Papyri and in drawings in the tombs. The healing skills were linked to the priesthood, to magicians and to certain families, but there was an organized school of medicine with a training programme. There were many different grades of specialists with a strictly demarcated area of practice, such as dentistry, bone setting, and abdominal diseases. The physicians, however, were instructed to be kind to their patients and not to abandon them, and the Papyri contain many maxims on ethical duties, such as 'not divulging secrets, nor looking at women in foreign households.' These may have been the forerunners of the Hippocratic Oath. There is some evidence that the Greek physicians visited Egypt and learnt from the Egyptians.

The Hippocratic Oath

It is often assumed that the Hippocratic Oath represented the normal practice of Greek doctors. However, careful research has shown that it originated from a small segment of Greek opinion, influenced by the Pythagorean philosophy and was not accepted by the majority. Medical writings from Hippocrates to Galen give evidence that Hippocratic principles were violated frequently. Indeed, it was quite common for doctors to put poison in the hands of their patients who intended to commit suicide, or to administer abortificients.

The Oath was probably written in the fourth century BC and it probably had no link with the famous Hippocrates of Cos. It was adopted by Christian Western Europe because its precepts coincided with the ethical principles of Christianity and Judaism. It was adopted by the Arabs and later by the scientists of the Renaissance because it also embodied their philosophies. Thus this famous oath can be described as a manifesto by a small group of ancient Greeks, which subsequently struck a cord in the minds of many physicians and seems to have linked the profession together across time and nation; but it is important to remind ourselves that it was the philosophy, or later, the religion, that formed the basis of the Oath, not vice versa. It is little wonder that the Oath has been largely forgotten in societies whose ethical bases have changed radically, where doctors break one of its clauses (e.g. abortion), and where some governments have passed laws encouraging the breaking of another (euthanasia).

The Oath's main principles can be summarized as *the duty*:

- To do no harm
- Not to assist suicide or administer euthanasia
- Not to cause abortion
- To refer patients for specialist treatment
- Not to abuse professional relationships, especially for sexual motives
- To keep the patient's confidences

These will be discussed in more detail in other sections of this book.

The quaint clauses about duties to the sons of one's teachers and the brotherhood of the profession must be seen in context. There were many charlatans practising at the time and it was important that only those who had the appropriate wisdom and knowledge should be practising medicine. To modern ears these phrases sound horribly like the blue-print for a nepotistic clique!

Other ancient writings

Other Greek writings about the duties of a physician have been discovered. One ancient poem was pieced together from fragments of stone discovered on the slopes of the Acropolis in Athens.

The Romans

There were famous Roman physicians and scientists, such as Galen, but Roman medicine was largely Greek medicine in a new context. Galen (AD 131–201) thought that the body was merely a vehicle for the soul and that its functions were therefore determined by God. Medicine was again closely related to religion. Although Galen was a very dogmatic teacher, very few new ideas were added by the Romans.

The Middle Ages

It is a common mistake to think of the Middle Ages in Europe as the dark ages of medicine and science, when ignorant quacks blundered from patient to patient. It is often seen as a quagmire of uncertainty between the clear thought and ethics of Greek medicine and the brilliant scientific research of the modern era. These generalizations are misleading and, whilst in the last section we saw that Greek medicine was not all practised by the Hippocratic ideal, in this section we will see that the Middle Ages were not all darkness. Certainly the Hippocratic ideal continued to have some influence, but there were writings about ethical matters which emanated from the monasteries of Northern Europe, written by St Jerôme amongst others, in the late fourth century AD. It must be remembered that medical practice and the care of the sick in Europe grew up closely linked with the Church, which was particularly involved in caring for the poor.

> The medieval physician, although he lacked skill and knowledge in the art and practice of medicine, in his humanity towards his patients and his desire to do the utmost to help them was equal to the best of our medical men today. These high ideals were held not by a few of these earlier doctors only but were the code of the profession.
>
> *Legacies* p. 204

Arabic and Islamic ethics

In a similar way, a treatise on the 'Practical Ethics of the Physician' was written in the eighth century for the Arab medical world, which sought to harmonize Islamic theology with Greek ethics. There was also some influence from the writings of Indian physicians and philosophers and translations from the ancient sources lead to a rapid development of Arabic science.

1600–1900 — the modern period

The Hippocratic Oath still had considerable influence at the end of Elizabethan times, but the following three hundred years were a period of enormous increase in knowledge and the development of scientific method. Starting in the wake of the Reformation in England and the liberation of thought from domination by the Roman Church, men of science were free to experiment. They could question the dogmas of both Galen's medicine and the Church. Many of the founders of the Royal Society in England were devout Christians but the freedom of thought created by this period led, in the eighteenth and nineteenth centuries, to other philosophies such as Evolutionary Humanism following Darwin's writings. There were, however, accounts of medical ethics written in the eighteenth century. The turmoil in the basis of ethics coincided with the founding of modern medicine. For example, anaesthesia and antiseptics were both discovered within a few years of the publication of Darwin's *On the origin of Species* (1859).

Another important development in this period was the rise of medical practice in North America, which, in turn, influenced medicine in Europe. American medicine grew up in the context of the westward migration and doctors would establish themselves behind the main front. The famous Mayo Clinic is one of the finest examples of the way opportunities were taken by an enterprising family of surgeons. However, the circumstances and relationships of practice were different from those left behind in Europe, and new ethical challenges appeared. Quite soon, ethical aspects were being

HISTORICAL PATHWAYS — II

MIDDLE AGES

ST. JERÔME

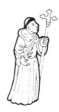

MODERN PERIOD

circa 1550   ELIZABETHAN

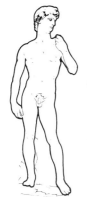

circa 1650   RENAISSANCE (ROYAL SOCIETY)

USA

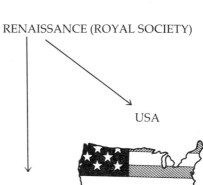

discussed, and in 1789, Professor Rush in Philadelphia gave a course of lectures on medical ethics. In the same year, Thomas Percival in Britain formulated his *Index of Medical Ethics*. It is interesting that many parts of the USA are far ahead of Britain in appointing staff members of medical schools to teach ethics and in establishing courses and departments for the subject.

1940 to the present day

The speed of change in medical practice of recent years has been staggering. One only has to consider what little could be done for the treatment of most diseases 50 years ago, to appreciate these changes. Antibiotics, hormone replacement therapy, vascular and heart surgery, not to mention transplantation and *in vitro* fertilization, have all been developed in this time. Traditional ethical values continued to be accepted in first part of the twentieth century, although the Christian foundation had been questioned and often abandoned, but it was the revelations of Hitler's atrocities involving doctors which really shook the medical world. It was realized that doctors *could* be put under extreme pressure by the State and *could* be involved in experiments which were evidently harmful to their coerced subjects. After the Nuremberg trials there was a re-statement of medical ethics, first as the Nuremberg Declaration and then as the World Medical Association's Declaration of Geneva (see p. 94). Rapidly, other codes and declarations followed: for research in patients (Helsinki), identification of death for organ transplantation (Sydney), and doctors and torture (Tokyo). This mushrooming of oaths and declarations reflected two trends:

1. The rapid change in medical practice. Whilst the doctor of the Middle Ages did all he could for his patients because he could do so little, the modern doctor can do so much and must ask whether there are times when it would be wiser and kinder to desist.
2. The worldwide links of medical practice and the different philosophies and religions that form the basis of ethics. Whilst one oath appeared to be sufficient for twenty centuries, at least six have appeared in the last forty years.

In the next chapter, we will consider who determines medical ethics today and explore the need for a system that can cope with changes over the next fifty years. These are likely to be even more rapid than they have been over the last half century.

HISTORICAL PATHWAYS — III

MODERN PERIOD (cont.)

Circa 1850

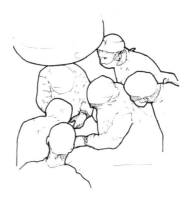

ANAESTHETICS
ANTISEPSIS

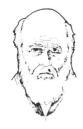

DARWIN

1940–PRESENT DAY

NUREMBERG

MODERN ETHICAL CODES

The Hippocratic Oath

I swear by Apollo the Physician and Asclepius and Hygieia and Panaceia and all the gods and goddesses, making them my witnesses, that I will fulfil according to my ability and judgement this oath and this covenant:

To hold him who has taught me this art as equal to my parents and to live my life in partnership with him, and if he is in need of money to give him a share of mine, and to regard his offspring as equal to my brothers in male lineage and to teach them this art — if they desire to learn it — without fee and covenant; to give a share of precepts and oral instruction and all the other learning to my sons and to sons of him who has instructed me and to pupils who have signed the covenant and have taken an oath according to the medical law, but to no one else.

I will apply dietetic measure for the benefit of the sick according to my ability and judgement; I will keep them from harm and injustice.

I will neither give a deadly drug to anybody if asked for it, nor will I make a suggestion to this effect. Similarly I will not give to a woman an abortive remedy. In purity and holiness I will guard my life and my art.

I will not use the knife, not even on sufferers from stone, but will withdraw in favor of such men as are engaged in this work.

Whatever houses I may visit, I will come for the benefit of the sick, remaining free of all intentional injustice, of all mischief and in particular of sexual relations with both female and male persons, be they free or slaves.

What I may see or hear in the course of the treatment or even outside the treatment in regard to the life of men, which on no account one must spread abroad, I will keep to myself holding such things shameful to be spoken about.

If I fulfil this oath and do not violate it, may it be granted to me to enjoy life and art, being honoured with fame among all men for all time to come; if I transgress it and swear falsely, may the opposite of all this be my lot.

References and Further Reading

Burns CR (ed) (1977). *Legacies in Ethics and Medicine*. Neal Watson Academic Publications Inc., New York.

Etziony MB (1973). *The Physician's Creed*. Charles C Thomas, Springfield, Illinois.

Review (1989). Contemporary lessons from Nazi medicine. Bulletin; **47**: 13–20, Institute of Medical Ethics.

Rhodes P (1985). *An Outline History of Medicine*. Butterworths, London.

3 Who makes the rules?

If a survey were taken of the informed, non-medical public, asking the question 'Who or what governs medical ethics in Britain today?' the answers would include: Parliament, the Hippocratic Oath, the British Medical Association, the Church, the General Medical Council, and the doctor's conscience. Some might be forgiven for thinking that the main influence was television! There is some truth in all these surmises and it is the purpose of this chapter to unravel the different influences on the practice of medicine today and to demonstrate the need for a clear framework for our thinking. We have already seen in the previous chapter how the Hippocratic Oath and the Christian faith provided guiding principles through the ages, but now Britain is a pluralistic society with many different philosophies and we have already rejected at least one of the Hippocratic ideals.

The General Medical Council (GMC)

The GMC was established under the Medical Act of 1858 and is a statutory body empowered by Parliament to govern the training of doctors and the practice of medicine. It keeps the medical Register and has the power, through its disciplinary committee, to suspend or strike a doctor off the register for serious professional misconduct. The GMC is made up of members of the profession and lay-members, and from time to time it gives ethical guidance on specific matters, particularly where these have been the subject of legal debate. A recent example is the guidance on *Professional Confidence: Treatment of Persons under 16* following the House of Lords' ruling in the Gillick case, which concerned the prescription of contraceptives to young girls. It was the GMC that recommended in 1967 that all medical schools should provide teaching in medical ethics. Not all schools have responded to this directive yet.

However, the GMC cannot govern the day-to-day decisions of doctors, and it cannot give detailed instructions for each situation. It is an overseeing and disciplinary body concerned with professional standards. Doctors cannot telephone the GMC each time they meet a problem; they need to learn to apply guidelines and think the problem through for themselves.

Other Councils

The United Kingdom Central Council for Nursing, Midwifery and Health Visiting, set up in 1979 to replace the General Nursing Council, is the controlling body for the nursing professions. In 1983, it issued a New Code of Professional Conduct and in 1987 a new document on confidentiality.

The Council for Professions Supplementary to Medicine performs a similar function for other healthcare workers, such as physiotherapists. The British Association of Social Workers has an ethical code but at present there is no compulsion for social workers to register with a disciplinary body.

Professional societies

The Medical Royal Colleges have issued ethical guidance (jointly and independently).

The British Medical Association (BMA), to which a majority of doctors belong (and a registered Trade Union since 1974), has been influential in formulating medical ethics over the years. It has a Central Ethical Committee and issues a *Handbook of Medical Ethics* which is updated from time to time, although the earlier versions were often dominated by matters of fees and etiquette. More recent editions have tackled the ethical dilemmas and a most welcome change in the latest copy (1988) is that it not only gives advice but outlines fully the philosophy and line of argument which gave rise to that advice. The BMA has also been active in advising and giving evidence to other bodies, such as the GMC and Royal Commissions. Of particular value is the BMA's recent concept of a checklist for the doctor to use in decision making (*Annual Report of Council*, 1987–88).

The Royal College of Nursing is a body very similar to the BMA in its ethical function for the nursing profession. It has been particularly clear in its guidance against strike action in recent disputes in the National Health Service. Doctors and nurses and other health professionals may be members of other Trade Unions but these, up to now, have been almost solely concerned with pay and conditions, rather than ethics.

The Defence Societies

The defence societies aim to provide legal and financial support by paying any damages and legal fees for doctors who are sued in the courts. It is compulsory to be a member of one of these societies in order to practise medicine within the British Health Service. Although they obviously have an interest in doctors behaving ethically, and they may provide guidance on individual situations, their role is legal rather than ethical in the more general sense.

The Law

The role of the law in medical ethics will be discussed in more detail later, but it must be remembered throughout these discussions that *a doctor is not above the law*. For example, the recent laws about access to, and confidentiality of, computerized records apply to medical records with only very special exceptions. A doctor has no legal right to break the speed limit or park on a double yellow line. If, however, these were absolutely necessary to help a patient in great need, the doctor would then be given leniency by the police, or in the courts. But the old trick of leaving a stethoscope on the back seat of the car, while parking illegally to buy some flowers for a perfectly fit mother-in-law, has been exposed for the deception it is!

The Employer

Most healthcare workers in Britain today are employed by the National Health Service (NHS) and although their contracts might be held at the local district or region, they are ultimately answerable to the Department of Health and the Minister of Health. To many people it might seem obvious that the employer should dictate the ethical behaviour of its employees and certainly the Department of Health does issue guidelines (e.g., for the testing of patients for HIV without consent); nevertheless, the employer can suspend or sack a doctor or nurse for gross unethical conduct. The employer holds this severe sanction against bad behaviour, but has little power actively to instil the best ethical behaviour. However, there is always the fear borne from experience in the past and in other countries that a monopoly employer, especially one under political control, could dictate to the doctor's conscience. At the present time in Britain, the employers do not usually interfere in the direct doctor/patient relationship, but financial considerations are begining to pose very large ethical problems for doctors, e.g., selecting which patients should be offered haemodialysis.

The World Medical Association (WMA)

The WMA has been responsible for a number of the Codes and Declarations that have been adopted worldwide. The WMA provides the forum for member associations to debate ethical issues and to try to reach universal principles of medical practice. It will be seen when these are discussed in more detail in Chapter 12, that some of them are very broad and non-specific. The WHO has no authority over the practice within member associations or states; but has an important advisory function in helping countries to set up their own indigenous organizations for ethical monitoring.

The need for pathways

New ethical dilemmas arrive at an alarming speed. It is easy to look back and see how historical codes shaped practice in the past, but now it is imperative that we devise a framework of thinking that can be applied to each new situation as soon as it presents. We also need pathways through the jungle of competing voices. The ethicist should aim to keep one step ahead of scientific progress. In the past, proverbs and aphorisms may have been sufficient because the problems were relatively simple. Are they sufficient for today? *Primum non nocere*, 'above all, do no harm' is one such aphorism derived from the Hippocratic Oath which has been quoted for years. At first sight, all would consent to such a worthy aim, but today when so many of our treatments have a potential for both harm and good, the doctor's skill in treating an individual is needed to ensure the good outweighs the harm. Modern cytotoxic anticancer drugs are a good example. They usually have marked side-effects, such as nausea and vomiting and hair loss. It is only justified to inflict these complications on a patient if there is a real chance of improving his quality, or length of life, significantly. If life expectancy is only increased by an average of 6 months at the price of 5 months of suffering earlier in the disease process, the treatment is not justified. The general public (and some lawyers) have not yet understood that any effective drug has a potential for unwanted side-effects (harm). Only oral sterile saline can be guaranteed to be harmless! Most modern surgical operations carry a small, but definite, mortality. If for a particular patient the chance of cure is very small, and the risk of postoperative death significant, then it would not be ethical to operate; but if the chances of cure or palliation were excellent, and the mortality risk low, it would be wrong *not* to operate for a serious condition. Nearly all modern ethical dilemmas involve a balancing act — the weighing up of factors that are in opposition to each other.
Despite their weaknesses, rules of thumb have an important

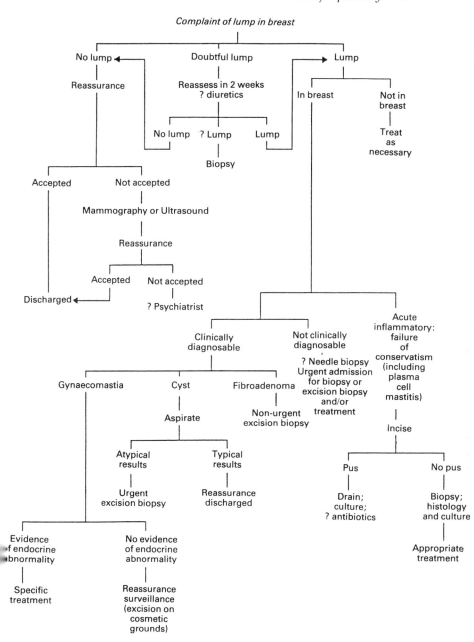

Figure 3.1   Pathways of surgical management (Reproduced by permission from Hobsley M. 1986 *Pathways in Surgical Management* 2nd Ed London: Edward Arnold)

place. It is not possible to derive every action from logical thought and analysis in a busy consulting room. Old proverbs such as 'honesty is the best policy' is at last being recognized as an important ethical rule in medicine! (See Chapter 14.) But in order to derive rules and actions, we must have pathways and algorithms. In everyday clinical medicine, a logical approach to diagnosis, investigation and treatment has become the pattern (see Fig. 3.2). If, for no other reason than economy, most doctors are turning against the 'fishing net' approach to investigating patients. This involves doing scores of tests and X-rays in a hope that one or two may prove positive. The pathways approach is to do the most discriminating simple tests first, and then, based on the results of these, follow one of the lines which may involve a few selected expensive tests. The same is true of ethical thinking; it is far more economical in time and thought to follow pathways than to cast out a net hoping to catch one or two 'fish' carrying ethical aphorisms in their mouths! The next chapter on analysing ethical dilemmas will develop this theme.

Who then makes the rules?

At the moment in Britain the answer is 'No one'; but many different groups have a hand in formulating ethical opinion. Certainly the decisions should not be left entirely to the medical and allied professions: lawyers, churchleaders and professional ethicists must

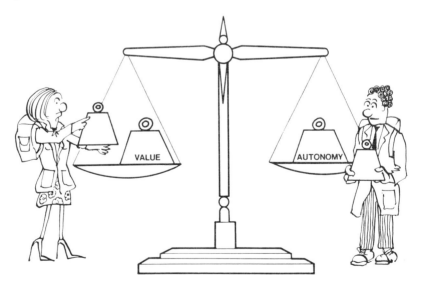

Figure 3.2   Many ethical decisions involve weighing of opposing factors

all play their part, but the person that is most often forgotten is the patient. It is important that all Hospital Ethical Committees have lay-members. However, it is the doctors and nurses who are at the bedside and it is often very difficult for others, who have not dealt with patients needing an urgent answer, to appreciate the pressure and emotional stress that these decisions entail. We will return to the question of 'who makes the rules' in the last chapter, but as Paul Ramsey has pointed out (in his paper 'The Nature of Medical Ethics', 1973), ethics are primarily concerned with *what* should be decided, rather than *who* should decide it.

References and Further Reading

British Medical Association (1988). *Annual Report of Council (1987–88)*.
British Medical Association (1988). *Philosophy and Practice of Medical Ethics*.
General Medical Council (1988). *Annual Report for 1987*.
Jackson D McG (1972). *Professional Ethics: who makes the rules?* Christian Medical Fellowship, London.
Ramsay P (1973). The nature of medical ethics. In *Teaching of Medical Ethics* (ed) Veatch RM. Hastings on Hudson, New York.
Ramsay P (1976). *The Patient as Person*. Yale University Press, Newhaven, Connecticut and London.

For regular reading on ethics
UK
The Journey of Medical Ethics
Bulletins published by Institute of Medical Ethics.

USA
Bioethics Quarterly published by the Northwest Institute of Ethics and Life Sciences.
Hasting Centre Reports published by the Institute of Society, Ethics and Life Sciences.

Addresses of professional organizations will be found in Appendix II.

4 Plotting the paths: analysing ethical dilemmas

Ethical decisions confront doctors and other healthcare professionals every day. Some are apparently trivial, whereas others seem insoluble; some are familiar and have well-established guidelines, others seem new and threatening. A dilemma, by definition, is a situation which requires a choice between two apparently equal alternatives and it is only by analysing the situation carefully that the real issues can be unravelled and adequate weighting given to each option. New ethical issues will continue to arise for as long as medicine progresses and human beings have moral codes, but the ingredients of the problem are usually the same as before, albeit in a different guise. The pathways are far more familiar than they appear at first sight and recognition of this fact goes a long way towards a solution.

These problems are analysed best by asking a number of key questions which ensure that the right path is taken at each crossroads. In this chapter, the questions will be presented and the different pathways described with examples, while in later chapters a variety of important issues will be analysed in this way.

Is there an ethical issue?

Once people have been made aware of medical ethics, it is tempting for them to see ethical issues in every clinical decision and to analyse each in great detail. This is both unnecessary and impractical and would bring our hospitals and surgeries to a standstill! Many everyday decisions are purely technical. For example, the decision about which antibiotic to give to a particular patient with an infection, is based on the sensitivity of the infecting organism and the spectrum of activity of the different antibiotics. It only becomes an *ethical* question when there is not enough money to buy the correct antibiotic or when there is an insufficient supply of the antibiotic to treat everybody with the infection. So, it is correct to say that it would be 'unethical' to use a very expensive antibiotic when a much cheaper one would be equally effective, and money so saved could be used to help another patient.

It is apparent, as pointed out in Chapter 1, that there is considerable confusion between ethics and etiquette. Ethics involve moral principles and values, whereas etiquette refers to customs and social conventions and is therefore less important and not so fundamental. The convention in Britain that a consultant will only see a patient who has been referred by his general practitioner is a matter of etiquette and does not apply in many other countries, whereas many of our ethical codes are accepted internationally. However, this etiquette has two important purposes: that of ensuring continuity of care through the general practitioner and ensuring that the patient sees the correct type of specialist for his or her particular needs. If left to his own devices the patient might refer himself inappropriately.

An apparently ethical issue may, in fact, be merely an emotional one. Although emotion should not be disparaged, sometimes an emotional dislike of a treatment can masquerade as an ethical principle. For example, if animal research is ethical at all, there is no ethical difference between using rats or cats; yet because cats are usually beloved household pets, their use is elevated to an ethical issue. Indeed, under the old legalization, an extra certificate was required from the Home Office for research involving dogs and cats.

The first part of the decision tree is summarized in Figure 4.1.

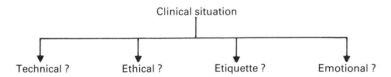

Figure 4.1

What are the ethical components?

We have already suggested that new ethical dilemmas do not often involve new ingredients but the same ingredient in a different form. Most of the medical ethical problems that face us are combinations of four general components:

1. **Aims** Our aims describe the ultimate purposes of medical care. For example, the WHO suggests that this should be 'to produce a complete sense of physical, mental and social wellbeing.'

2.   **Value**   This assesses the worth of human life, and relative value at different stages of development. For example, does value diminish with (old) age, and is it equally present in the immature or malformed? Why do we regard human life as worth more than other animal life?

3.   **Autonomy**   Autonomy considers the freedom to determine one's own actions and behaviour, particularly when the decision concerns one's own body, and is illustrated by the importance of the patient's consent before a surgical operation. It also includes a debate about one individual imposing his moral principles on another, for example, in refusing or agreeing to abortion.

4.   **Truth**   Truth concerns the telling of the truth to the patient about her illness but also includes confidentiality and promise-keeping, such as not giving information to a third party without the patient's agreement.

Each of these ethical components will be discussed in more detail in the following chapters. Some situations relate to only one of these components, while others involve a combination of two or three. For example, the worldwide distribution of resources involves both aims and values. First, we must ask what medicine is trying to achieve. Is it the greatest good to the greatest number, spreading the resources as evenly and widely as possible? Or should the distribution be selective to particular areas of need, involving a decision about the relative value of people of different races, ages or social backgrounds?

When we consider the problem of research on patients, three ethical pillars are linked: value, autonomy and truth. Value is involved because the value of the patient undergoing, say, a new treatment, is being compared with the value of society (patients as a whole) who may benefit from the results of the research. Autonomy is relevant because the patient must have the right to decide, voluntarily and without pressure, whether to take part in the experimental study. Finally, truth is involved, because of the importance of informed consent and the question of how much should be explained to the patient. As a further example, the vexed question of how much to tell a patient with cancer, is based on the twin ethical pillars of truth and autonomy: the doctor not misleading the patient and the patient having the right (only if she wishes) to make decisions about her own treatment.

The whole abortion debate centres on the value of the fetus at different stages of its development and the mother's right to decide (autonomy).

Recently, the problem of AIDS (Acquired Immune Deficiency Syndrome) has burst upon the scene and difficult ethical problems have to be faced. But has AIDS produced any *new* ethical problems?

Again, the main elements are truth and autonomy, illustrated by the importance of confidentiality when the doctor knows a patient is HIV-positive, the question of whether or not to test for HIV without the patient's consent (even if the knowledge obtained could protect others), and whether society should impose a certain code of sexual behaviour on patients to prevent the spread of the disease (autonomy).

The second phase of analysis is shown in Figure 4.2.

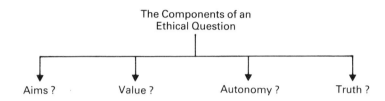

Figure 4.2

What are the ethical principles?

Having decided on the main components of the problem, we must now look at them in more detail and extract the principles. At first sight, it might seem that there is little difference between a component and a principle but there is indeed an important distinction. It is linked to the definition of medical ethics in Chapter 1, where ethics were referred to as 'obligations'. Components are merely the different arenas of ethical debate that give no guidance and no obligation. Principles are the ethical obligations which govern decision-making. Ethical principles may be *general* or *specific*. Here are some examples of such principles:

In the area of aims of health care, the *general* ethical principle might be that of justice and a *specific* principle that health care should be distributed to all according to need.

In the realm of value, the *general* ethical principle might be the very high value of human life and the *specific* principles that (1) it should be respected from conception to death, and (2) that its value is the same, irrespective of nationality, sex, colour and religion.

In the realm of *autonomy*, the *general* principle might be that each human being has a right to make decisions that will affect his own destiny and a *specific* principle, that he should have autonomy in deciding whether or not to consent to an operation.

In the realm of truth, the *general* principle is that truth is right and good and therefore the *specific* principle is that to tell lies to patients about their illness is wrong.

It is important to consolidate somewhat abstract concepts such as justice and truth into definite statements and proposals. It is at this level of ethical statements that the codes may be helpful because they put general principles into statements and promises (*see* Chapter 12). In the Hippocratic Oath 'I will neither give a deadly drug . . .' is a specific statement arising from the principle of the utmost respect for human life. In a few cases, the law is specific enough to be helpful in establishing statements, but its function is largely a 'perimeter fence' to prevent gross departures from ethical behaviour. For example, the law will say 'You shall not murder' but this is a long way from the notion of utmost respect for human life (this is discussed further in Chapter 13). We may adopt the general ethical principle mentioned above that 'telling the truth is right and good' and the specific principle or statement 'I will not tell lies to my patient'. However, in order to appreciate the force of this statement, we need to ask why telling lies is wrong and this leads us back to the basis of our ethics — theistic and humanistic — the nature of God and the nature of man.

These deductions are summarized in Figure 4.3.

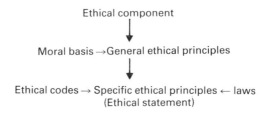

Figure 4.3

Moral bases

The basis of ethics not only undergirds and establishes the principles, but also influences the weighting given to each when there is a conflict between them. For a pure teleologist without a basis in this sense, the weighting of the different actions will be decided by the likely consequences (*see* Figure 4.7), but for the deontologist, the strength of the principle will be determined by the certainty of the basis and the sanctions behind it. This will be discussed further in Chapter 5. It is important to note here, however, that theistic and atheistic morals can sometimes produce the same principles and sometimes very different principles. Figure 4.4 shows this stage of the decision-making in diagrammatic form.

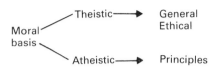

Figure 4.4

Ethical principles in conflict

The major problem with ethical decisions, and by which they become dilemmas, is that two ethical principles or obligations appear to conflict with each other. These may be within the same component or between different components. For example, within the field of autonomy, there may be a direct conflict between the autonomy of two people — the doctor and the patient. Alternatively, the conflict may be between two different components, e.g., the value of the fetus against the autonomy of the mother. The relative weight put on one or another of the principles determines the outcome. One gynaecologist might decide that the value of the fetus is so minimal that abortion decisions should be based on autonomy alone, and it is up to the mother to decide. He will then advise her purely on the physical and emotional consequences to her of one or other course of action. But another gynaecologist will argue that this autonomy must be limited and even subordinated to the principle of human value. A third gynaecologist might go even further and consider that fetal value is the overriding principle, that the mother should have very little say in the matter and her autonomy overruled. (Absolutes — "through ways")

The decision about conflicting principles is outlined in Fig. 4.5.

The local factors

A conflict of two equally strong ethical principles can only be resolved by one taking absolute priority, local factors favouring one or the other or both being honoured by the way the study is designed or the situation handled (by 'local' factors I am referring to the special details of the particular situation).

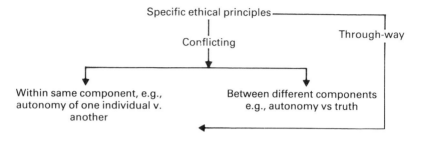

Figure 4.5

We may have two ethical principles which appear to conflict, such as a research project in which there is a conflict between the patient's autonomy and the good of many other people with a serious disease. Some moral philosophies, such as Marxism, would accept the principle that an individual's wellbeing may often be subordinated to the welfare of society as a whole. The conflict is then resolved. However, if a moral basis stresses the great value of the individual as well as the value of society as a whole, there is a real problem of priority. We must then ask whether, in this particular situation, there are any other factors which give weight to one or the other. This has been well established, for example, with certain infectious diseases, where the individual's right to refuse treatment is subordinated (in law) to the welfare of all, because the consequences are so severe. On the other hand, in an experiment to investigate some basic human function or process, a normal volunteer's autonomy is respected above all else.

Lest it should be assumed that ethical arguments always have to end in irreconcilable conflict, very often the design of a study or the

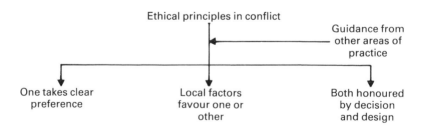

Figure 4.6

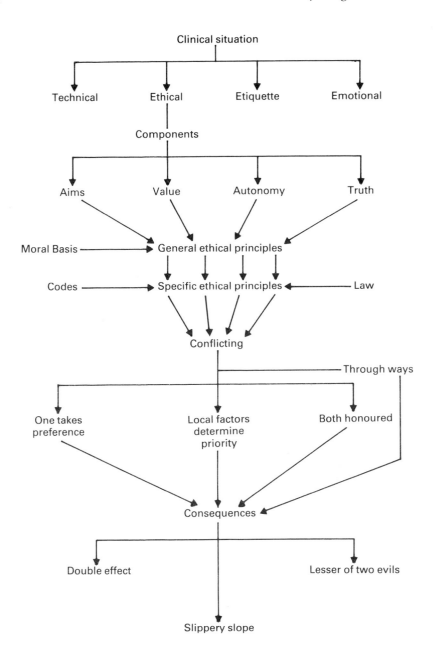

Figure 4.7

way questions are asked can accommodate both ethical principles and so resolve the conflict. This is true of telling patients they have cancer. The way they are told can minimize distress, maintain the doctor/patient relationship, give the patient maximum involvement in discussions about her illness (autonomy) and convey the truth. Further examples will be given in later chapters, but the possible ways of resolving ethical conflicts are outlined in Figure 4.6.

In summary, the overall decision tree (algorithm) for analysing practical ethical problems and resolving them from the *standpoint of ethical principles* is shown in Figure 4.7. For those whose ethics are not as much based on principles as on consequences, the algorithm is a little different. (Consequences are discussed in Chapter 11) The early part of the analysis is the same (Figures 4.1 and 4.2) but then the middle part is left out (Figures 4.3, 4.4 and 4.5). The possible decisions are outlined and possible consequences of each are extrapolated. A scoring is then given to each of the consequences and, either by the criterion of the 'greatest good for the greatest number' or the criterion of 'the greater good for one individual compared with another', the decision is made. The problem comes when we try to decide what is 'good'.

5 The starting points: the basis of ethics

The study of medical ethics is the study of values in the care of sick people and values must be derived from somewhere or someone. A group of health professionals must also have an obligation to apply what is good and right. The two basic questions in medical ethics are therefore these:

1. What is the source of values? How do we know what is right and good?

2. Where does a sense of obligation come from? Why should we do what is right and good, and to whom are we responsible for our decisions and actions?

Plato, on the one hand, defined moral good as a harmony of all the virtues under the rule of reason, these virtues existing independently of any person. But he made the naive assumption that those who know what is good will love and desire it. Jean-Paul Sartre on the other hand, being an atheistic existentialist, thought that values are entirely man-made and any obligation is entirely self-imposed. But do human beings even keep to their own self-made rules? The history of New Year resolutions is not encouraging! The next few sections of this book will show briefly how different religions and philosophies answer these questions.

The prevailing philosophy in Britain today is impossible to define because it is an amalgamation of many views. Three-quarters of the population say they believe in a God of some kind, but less than 10 per cent go to church. Thirty five years ago, science was God, but its failure to produce good without bad, led to disillusionment and to the young people of the 1960s seeking out mystical experiences in the East. Whatever people say in newspaper surveys about their religious views, in practice, the prevailing mood is agnostic, if not atheistic, spiced with the vague memory of a religious ethic inherited from grandparents. Within the medical profession, values have changed more slowly than in the rest of society, but only a minority of students entering medicine would be able to explain why they believed what they believed about moral matters. The main change in thought that has influenced the academic world over the last hundred years is atheistic humanism (naturalism). As Baroness Wootton writes (qv):

> Nothing perhaps separates this century from its immediate predecessor as the loss amongst educated men and women of conviction of the literal truth of the basic dogmas of the Christian religion and of the certainty of individual survival after death. As a result of this loss, a tremendous, though generally silent, shift has occurred in the basis of morality. We ask no longer what is pleasing to God, but what is good for man.

Let us then start with a brief review of atheistic world views.

Atheistic world views

The belief that unites atheistic views is that God does not exist; therefore values and obligations cannot be derived from outside this world. They must come from references to man himself. There is no creator and the humanist finds

> . . . insufficient evidence for belief in the existence of a supernatural
> *Humanist Manifesto*, II: 1973

Scientific humanism

This philosophy started at the beginning of the last century, although its seeds were sown many years before and it was given great impetus by Darwin's discoveries as interpreted by Thomas Henry Huxley. In this century scientific humanism has been championed by Bertrand Russell, GE Moore and Sir Julian Huxley, amongst others. In outline, it states that:

* Matter is all that there is
* The cosmos exists in a closed system of cause and effect
* Personality is a function of physiochemical interrelations
* There is no life after death.

A few quotations will illustrate these points:

> As far as we know the total personality is a function of the biological organism transacting in a social and cultural context
> *Humanist Manifesto* II.

> Organic evolution is a process entirely materialistic in its origin and operation
> *G G Simpson*

How then does humanism answer the two questions we posed at the beginning of the chapter? The answer of *Humanist Manifesto II* (qv) to the source of values is this:

> We affirm that moral values derive their source from human experience, ethics are autonomous and situational, needing no theological or ideological sanction. Ethics stem from human need and interest.

A thorough-going evolutionist would go further and say that good is what promotes the survival and improvement of the human *species* as opposed to the individual.

The humanist answer to the question of obligation is that it is derived from the sense of values in the environment and general obligation to the human race. There is no logical reason for caring for the handicapped in society except in so far this action reflects an opinion of man and the value of mankind as a whole. The humanist is responsible to man alone. He recognizes that man is not yet good but relies on a gradual evolutionary improvement to perfect man's moral character as well as his body.

Marxism (dialectical materialism)

A large proportion of the world is under the influence of Marxism and so it is relevant to look at its ethics. There is no doubt that Marxism shares humanism's atheism. It is primarily an economic system which governs all human activity, so a value of an action or person is derived from its economic value or value to society. Initially this was to a particular class in society but later to society as a whole when this became 'classless'. A sense of obligation is derived from dedication to the party and will of the people. There is no logical reason in this system for keeping alive anyone who is handicapped and cannot contribute to society. The Marxist is responsible to the Party, his comrades and the State.

Atheistic existentialism

This movement is associated with the names of Kierkegaard, Sartre and others and shares many of the basic tenets of humanism that God does not exist and that the cosmos is a uniformity of cause and effect in a closed system. However, existentialists stress a subjective world of mind and awareness in which man is free and which is not influenced by science and logic. Therefore, value is created just by someone choosing that course of action. Sartre writes:

> . . . To choose to do this or that is to affirm at the same level the value of what we choose, because we can never choose evil, we always choose the good.

There is no sense of obligation because there are no external reference points and each person is free to choose for himself. The existentialist is responsible to no one but his own subjective self. If all doctors were thorough-going existentialists, it would be very difficult to establish a code of ethics! But a watered down existentialist attitude pervades medicine today. 'We will just have to treat every case on its merits' is a very common end to a discussion on medical ethics, implying that if we do our best in all honesty, that will make the decision right.

Utilitarianism

This philosophy championed by John Stuart Mill and Jeremy Bentham, amongst others, judges the value of an action in terms of its consequences (*see* p. 45) — the greatest good for the greatest number. Jeremy Bentham (whose clothed waxed body still adorns the corridor of University College, London) was a hedonist which means that, for him, good was pleasure. The problem is to decide what sort of pleasure: mental, physical, or aesthetic? Mill solved the problems by grading the pleasures into higher (intellectual) and lower (physical). The sense of obligation comes from a desire to give pleasure to others or oneself. The utilitarian is responsible to the 'general good'. We might ask what happens to minority rights. The effects of utilitarianism will be considered further in Chapter 7.

This brief outline summarizes the essence of each world view, but there are obviously many variations on each theme. Books have been written on each and can be studied in more detail, if required. It is hoped that enough detail has been given to show the varying starting points of different atheistic philosophies, let alone their fundamentally different approaches, from the theistic philosophies to be outlined in the next section.

Theistic moral systems

These all have in common a reference to a supernatural being (God) who, in various ways, has revealed His will and system of values. There is an external set of standards and a sense of obligation comes from the acceptance of God's authority and will.

Judaism

Judaism has had a considerable influence on medical ethics throughout history, both in its own right and through Christianity. Jews believe that God is not only the creator of an ordered world but also involved in it. The universe is not a closed system and God can and does influence what goes on. He has made His values known, especially through the Ten Commandments (Exodus: 20), but also through many other instructions written down by the Prophets. Good is what agrees with God's character. The sense of obligation and responsiblity is to a just and holy God who has made man 'estate manager' of the rest of creation.

> When I consider your heavens, the work of your fingers, the moon and stars, which you have set in place, what is man that you are mindful of him, the son of man that you care for him? . . . You made him ruler over the works of your hands; you put everything under his feet
>
> The Bible, Psalm 8.

Jews would also point out that God's laws are not capricious but are made for man's benefit (e.g., the sound public health laws in the book of Leviticus). There is, in each person, an immortal soul, which represents his true self, and which survives death. God rewards or punishes people according to their deeds and so keeping observances and customs is very important for the Jew.

Christianity

Christianity accepts the Jewish revelations of God and its value system but goes one important stage further. Christians believe that God revealed His will supremely by Jesus Christ, who was God Himself in human form.

> The Word became flesh and lived for a while among us. We have seen his glory, the glory of the one and only Son, who came from the Father, full of grace and truth.
>
> The Bible, John 1:14

He not only taught God's moral standards, e.g., in the Sermon on the Mount (Matthew: 4 and 5) but showed them, perfectly, by the way He lived. So, Christians claim they are not just trying to obey a set of difficult moral rules but following a person, and when they want to know how much God values a blind beggar or a patient with leprosy, they see how Jesus handled the situation. Good is what corresponds to God's character and will and the ultimate motive is self-sacrificing love.

> Love is patient, love is kind. It does not envy, it does not boast, it is not proud. It is not rude, it is not self-seeking, it is not easily angered, it keeps no record of wrongs. Love does not delight in evil but rejoices with the truth
>
> The Bible, 1 Corinthians: 4–7

So Christians would point out that motivation matters, and they talk about Christ's spirit motivating them and helping them to do what is right. Death is not the extinction of personality, but the gateway to a new and better life for those who believe. Both Jews and Christians recognize that people are imperfect and fail to live up to their high ethical standards. In fact, without God's help, they believe that there is a natural human tendency to do evil. Unlike humanists, they do not see that man will naturally improve his moral stature. However, it is a caricature of both the Jewish and Christian view of God to picture Him as a bearded vengeful old man in the sky, waiting to catch people out whenever they put a foot wrong. Forgiveness, because of the death and resurrection of Christ, is the keystone of Christianity.

There are two main traditions in Christianity which affect ethical discussion. The Roman Catholics put great stress on the authority of the Pope and the Church in the interpretation of the Bible and so have a more uniform and strict ethical code, e.g., on abortion and contraception. They also emphasize the role of *natural law* — that is, that general moral laws can be deduced even by non-Christians from observation of God's creation. Protestants, on the other hand, have tended to leave the interpretation and application of biblical teaching to the individual and his own conscience, so there is more variation in their ethical views (e.g., on abortion) although nearly all Protestants would see abortion as a lesser of two evils, rather than good.

Islam

Islam is similar to Judaism and Christianity in its view of one God, but Muslims believe that Mohammed and the Koran rather than Christ and the Bible are the final revelation from God (Allah) and that the model behaviour of Mohammed is the example to follow. Many of the virtues and values are the same as those in the other main religions — honesty, humility, charity and kindness etc., and there are strict laws on many different aspects of life. In the first four to five centuries of Islam, many of the doctors were, in fact, Jews and Christians and so the religious influence on medicine was mixed. There is a strong sense of fatalism in Islam, in that a person's life events are determined by Allah and nothing can be done to alter them. Islamic, like Greek, medical ethics were particularly concerned with the profession rather than the patients because of the many charlatans practising at the time.

Other religions and philosophies

Deism

Differs from theistic religions such as Christianity in that deists believe in a God who started the world but who then withdrew and left it to run itself. Man can find out what God is like by studying the universe and deducing its rules and values, rather than by any special revelation. Thus, what is seen in the universal laws of nature is right. A sense of obligation is in a general sense to God and nature but there is no specific responsibility to a person. This view, with its variations, is probably the most common background philosophy of British doctors today.

Hinduism

Hinduism is a mixture of faiths and has many different branches. God is thought of as being present in everything and every place. Men can find God by dedicating work to Him, by prayer and love, and by contemplation — helped by such excercises as Yoga. Until a man finds the ultimate reality, he is reincarnated again and again, and everything in this world is only illusion. Certain animals are sacred, and the caste system is obviously important when considering the relative value of different people in society. In ancient writings, the doctor is forbidden to treat certain types of people, including patients with incurable diseases.

Buddhism

Buddhists follow the teaching of the Buddha and do not worship God. Their aim is to attain Nirvana which is a state of perfect peace and freedom from suffering. The Buddha was greatly influenced as a young man by witnessing suffering, and he aimed to help his fellow man. As Buddhists believe in the reincarnation of the soul into many different kinds of animal they have the profoundest respect for all life and strict Buddhist will not even kill a mosquito.

Astrology

Guidance through omens in the stars has a long history from ancient Egypt through the Greeks and Romans to the present day. In the last twenty-five years, reliance on horoscopes has increased enormously in Britain, and now they are even computerized! Many people probably follow their stars in a light-hearted manner but some take them very seriously. They have a bearing on ethics in that a person may believe she cannot help her temperament, or behaviour, because 'she is made like that' and is under the impersonal influence of external forces. There is, therefore, little sense of obligation or responsibility to anyone else.

This is, necessarily a very brief review and readers are strongly encouraged to read for themselves the source of material that is listed below. However, in the chapters that follow, reference will be made to the way these different world views work out in practice.

References and Further Reading

Bentham J (1789). *An Introduction to the Principles of Morals and Legislation.* Methuen, London.
Biblical References from *The Bible: New International Version* (1989). Hodder and Stoughton, London.
Holmes AF (1984). *Ethics: Approaching Moral Decisions.* Inter-Varsity Press, Illinois and Leicester.
Humanist Manifestos I and II. Prometheus Books, New York. (Manifesto II is also published in *The Humanist* (1973).)
Jakobovitz I (1975). *Jewish Medical Ethics* (2nd edn.). Block, New York.
Mill JS (1863). *Utilitarianism* (ed) Warnick M (1979). Fount paperbacks, London.
Sartre J-P (1947). *Existentialism and Humanism*, translated by Mairet P (1973). Eyre Methuen, London.
Simpson GG (1951). *The Meaning of Revolution.* Mentor Books, New York.
Wilkinson J (1988). *Christian Ethics in Health Care.* Handsel Press, Edinburgh.
Wooton, Baroness (1961). In *The Humanist Frame* (ed) Sir Julian Huxley. George Allen and Unwin, London.

See Also
Entries under philosopher's names in *A Dictionary of Philosophy* (see chapter 1).
Entries under various religions and philosophies in *A Dictionary of Medical Ethics* (see chapter 1).
Sire JW (1977). *The Universe Next Door: a guide to world views.* Inter-Varsity Press, Leicester.

6 Ethical component I: the aims of medical care

What is the aim of modern medicine? What are we trying to achieve? This may seem a silly question with an obvious answer: 'To cure ill patients, or prevent them becoming ill, of course!' But the question is more complicated than it seems and is very rarely asked, although billions of pounds are poured into the National Health Service each year. The answer, in terms of immediate priorities, may be very different in Japan from that in a developing African country, where a clean water supply is a most urgent need. But the question about overall aims and strategy still remains. To unravel this problem it will be helpful to discuss some well-known maxims which are often quoted in this context.

'The greatest good for the greatest number'

We have already referred to this famous utilitarian motto in Chapter 5. It seems, at first sight, to be uncontroversial but it raises socially important questions: Who decides what is good? We have already seen that Mill and Bentham could not agree on what pleasures were the most pleasurable! Bentham proposed a hedonic calculus in which for each line of action (or treatment) the pleasure can be quantified in terms of its intensity, duration, certainty or uncertainty, nearness or remoteness, freedom from pain and how many people are affected. In clinical decisions we often do a similar sort of predictive assessment of a patient's wellbeing — for example, when we try to assess the likely outcome with and without a certain operation. But it is often difficult to quantify wellbeing in any meaningful way, whereas parameters such as length of life and closeness of death are far easier to handle. The other problem is how the 'greatest number' is calculated. Is this an *average* wellbeing or a maximum? If it is an average, then the very inequalities which many doctors are trying to eliminate are concealed. If medical care is spread too thinly, no one will benefit; so the greatest good conflicts with the greatest number. Does one define an arbitrary moderate level of health and then try to get as many people as possible to that level? The United Nations has decided that access to a minimum degree of health care is a basic human right. The WHO slogan 'Health for all by the Year 2000' is a laudable ideal but raises the question of what we mean by health, which will be discussed in more detail below. Access to health *care* for all is a more meaningful and realistic aim.

'Above all, do no harm'

This has been used as a general aim for hundreds of years but its inadequacy as a blueprint for modern medicine is clear. Obviously, it is important that doctors do no intentional harm without a very great chance of greater benefit; but this policy is negative. It could encourage health workers to do nothing rather than risk harming the patient, and in so doing do a greater harm by leaving him untreated. More important, is the corollary of 'doing no harm', i.e., 'doing good' — the principle of *beneficence*.

Beneficence

The underlying basis for the trust that a patient has for you, his doctor, is that you will always act in his best interests — for his benefit. Beneficence means that a doctor will do what is good for the patient, not what is good for the doctor. It is particularly relevant in a private system of medical care where unnecessary operations can easily be done when the fees are very high. In the USA, hospitals have set up Tissue Committees to ensure that too many normal appendices and uteri are not being removed. Removing normal organs may not do the patient much harm, but certainly does not do him any good. Some doctors make the diagnosis of 'chronic remunerative appendicitis!' In State medicine, the temptations are different when 'failure to do good' becomes the problem. The commonest reason for referral to the Disciplinary Committee of the GMC is 'Disregard of Professional reponsibilities to patients.' The problem, therefore, is doing harm by neglect rather than by direct action.

'To cure sometimes, to relieve often, to comfort always'

This famous quotation from the fifteenth century was inscribed on the Statue of Dr EL Trudeau, the American pioneer in the treatment of tuberculosis. It was a realistic assessment of the aims of medical care in its time. Has this now changed, with all the new modern scientific discoveries? Is it too low an aim? In fact, nothing very much has changed. Modern medicine has done nothing to increase the life span of human beings, but has helped very many people to reach a ripe old age (as our NHS has begun to realize). We still cure relatively few illnesses. Of the common operations, appendicectomy cures appendicitis but even hernia repairs and vagotomies for duodenal ulcers have a recognized recurrence rate. Most vascular surgery is palliative and the underlying disease is unaffected, only one or two complications being treated by the operation. Some cancers are cured but many more are only relieved. Far more people have their symptoms improved than they did years ago but often we have treated one group of diseases, e.g., infections, to find them replaced in later life by degenerative and malignant conditions. The important question, especially when treating cancer, is when the healthcare team must change from a 'curing mode' to a 'relieving mode' (to use modern jargon). Treatment of symptoms (palliation) is very worthwhile and just as much part of treatment as an attempted cure but modern scientific medicine has been slow to realize this. Recently, consultant appointments in palliative medicine have at last given official approval to this concept.

However, our underlying philosophies (Chapter 5) make an important contribution here. The humanist could justifiably ask 'What is the point of merely palliating a patient with an incurable painful illness? Her life has no value (see below) and it should be ended to save suffering and expense.' Many people, on the other hand, have too high an expectation of modern scientific medicine. It is not, and never will be, the answer to all society's problems, and in the end its plans will always be frustrated by death; but it can *improve* people's lives tremendously. Sir Peter Medawar in his book, *Advice to a Young Scientist*, contrasts scientific messianism (science is the answer to all our problems) with scientific meliorism (science can help to improve many problems). It is important to put science in its rightful place!

'Prolong life at all costs'

This is often quoted as an aim for medical care, but it is difficult to find where it actually originated. It seems to be a deduction from the biblical command 'not to kill' and the Hippocratic injunction to 'keep patients from harm'. There would be few doctors today who would support this as the overriding aim of modern medicine. Certainly, Christian teaching is that the *quality* of life is as important as its *length* and for those who believe in heaven, death is not the worst thing that can happen. The distinction between prolonging life by *ordinary* and *extraordinary* means is well established in ethical thinking and was given the blessing of Pope Pius the XII in 1957. However, respect for life does not necessarily imply prolonging it at all costs. The Declaration of Geneva uses the word 'respect' when it says 'I will maintain the utmost respect for human life from the time of conception.' Indeed, one of the arguments of those supporting voluntary euthanasia is that their respect for life makes them unable to tolerate a slow, painful, lingering death. The *utmost* respect for life implies that this respect is a very high order and very few, if any, other principles should override it. This will be discussed in more detail in Chapter 7.

'To restore patients to health'

Surely no one can argue with this aim! But it all depends on what we mean by health. Health has the connotation of wholeness which, in turn, implies not only the proper functioning of each system, but its correct integration in a 'whole person'. This is very topical in view of the increased interest in holistic medicine and the rejection of scientific medicine's preoccupation with the physical.

The WHO defines health as 'a complete sense of physical, mental and social wellbeing' which sounds grand. But is 'a complete sense of social wellbeing' one car or two, a washing machine, a colour television or none of these? Sometimes we have to choose between mental and physical wellbeing because attempts to produce physical improvement, e.g., in a spina bifida child, is bought at the expense of severe mental stress and stunted emotional development caused by many visits to hospital for repeated operations. The WHO definition, by using the words 'sense', suggests that freedom from stress of any kind is the aim of health care. However, no one will develop either physically or mentally or emotionally without the right amount of challenge and stress. Is virtue more important than pleasure as Kant and other philosophers have maintained? This is not to conclude that pain and suffering are good, but many religious people and some atheists would maintain that stress and suffering can be turned to a greater good if handled positively. Some would like to add the word 'spiritual wellbeing' to the definition but this might be considered to be outside the immediate brief of medical care itself. The other great weakness of this definition is that a sense of wellbeing is very subjective and depends on previous experience. It could be argued that the way to fulfil this idea of health is to prevent people knowing anything better than their present situation! Having said all that, the WHO definition must be welcomed for its stress on the wholeness and integration of the human being.

What is normal health?

'There is no such thing as a healthy person, only one who has been inadequately investigated!' — a Professor of Medicine is supposed to have said. This cynical view does raise the problem of how we tell when our patient has been restored to health; is there a norm or an ideal? Certainly we can describe normal physiology in terms of a range of normal values, such as the body temperature and the electrolytes in the blood. But the normal is much more difficult to define and the variation far wider, when we consider mental health and social relationships. Someone might well ask whether a paralysed person in a wheelchair, who is mentally alert and spiritually radiant is more or less healthy than a professional boxer who is superbly fit, physically, but mentally very dull and spiritually dead! (For a moving autobiography of a girl suddenly paralysed in her teens *see Joni,* Further Reading.) Perhaps the old public school motto *Mens sana in corpore sano* — 'a sound mind in a sound body' is, after all, the aim of medical care!

Should medicine aim to alter normal physiology?

Up until recently, this has not been an issue because it was not often possible. However, the regular use of the contraceptive pill was the first time that normal hormonal physiology was altered long-term for millions of people. Most people today would see this as a justifiable (though not ideal) interference with normal function, but this may be the thin edge of the wedge. What about improving the human species, guiding the evolutionary process and producing a superman? George Bernard Shaw's reply to the dancer, Isadora Duncan, is well known. When Miss Duncan suggested that they should have children, who could then inherit a combination of her body and his brains, Shaw is supposed to have replied 'But supposing our children had my body and your brains!' However, before the end of World War II, Hitler had started to breed his super race by mating specially chosen SS officers with the most beautiful girls in Germany. We are now forced back to the logical effects of the different philosophies discussed in Chapter 5. To Hitler, who embraced the evolutionary model of the survival of the fittest and applied it to different races of human beings, many of his actions were at least consistent with his philosophy. We will turn again to the question of the limits of medicine when we look at the question of fetal tissue transplantation (Chapter 18).

The importance of purpose

The problem with much of our modern scientific medicine is that it is orientated towards procedures and techniques rather than towards patients and purposes. We develop a new technique and then see how we can use it rather than have an overall strategy for health care. Highly prestigious and expensive buildings so often take the money away from prevention of illness in both developing and developed countries. The new awareness of the effect of diet and lifestyle has drawn attention again to the importance of prevention, but the way our health systems are usually financed does not encourage preventative medicine. However, to give credit where it is due, the world wide immunization programmes have been an outstanding success, not least in eradicating smallpox from the face of the earth and, in Britain, almost eliminating diphtheria, polio, tetanus and whooping cough. But to return to the idea of purpose, perhaps we can define the aims of medical care as helping the patient to realize his or her full potential — physical, mental, social and spiritual (for those who wish to include it). This allows for the difference in potential between different patients and the fact that for some there is no chance of getting one function back (e.g., the use of their legs) but the rest of their bodies and their mental and emotional powers can be restored. For others, it must be admitted that their mental capacity is very limited but it can, at least, be developed to its full potential. This concept gets us away from an arbitrary level for a norm of healthiness.

When selection has to be made

When we come to discuss the allocation of resources, there is no easy answer and there are many compounding factors such as political obstruction and war. It is incumbent upon all involved in health, to obtain accurate facts of the cost-effectiveness of different policies. However, choice will always have to be made and priorities determined. Left to a free market economy, the wealthy and those of high social status will get the best care. This again takes us back to the basic philosophies. Is this right? For the survival of the fittest and improvement of the race, it may be. On the other hand, the Judaeo–Christian emphasis has always been on helping the poor and those who *cannot* help themselves. These can often be distinguished from those who *will* not help themselves. Christians are expected to have compassion, even on those who have brought the illness on themselves. (These form a large proportion of patients in our hospitals today, if the effects of smoking, overeating, alcohol abuse, and sexual irresponsibility are all combined.) The history of medical care in Europe and many tropical countries has been guided by these principles and the obligation of compassion.

References and Further Reading

Duggan JM (1989). Resource allocation and bioethics. *Lancet*; **i**: 772–3.

Eareckson J (1976). *Joni*. Pickering and Inglis, London and Glasgow.

Illich I (1976). *Limits to Medicine: medical nemesis, the expropriation of health.* Marion Bogars, London.

Kennedy IM (1981). *The Unmasking of Medicine.* George Allen and Unwin, London.

Medawar PB (1979). *Advice to a Young Scientist.* Harper and Row, New York.

7 Ethical component II: the value of human life

In Britain we are used to putting a high value on human life. It was not long ago that the punishment for murder was quite different in quality, not just degree, from that for all other crimes. We mobilize the rescue services just as urgently when one person is stranded on a mountainside, as when 20 people are. Wherein does this value lie? Why do we value people whom we may never have met and know nothing about, just because they are human beings? The value that we place on an *animal* depends on three things, 1. its rarity, 2. its economic value, and 3. its aesthetic value. We put a very high value on the giant panda because it is very rare and it looks quaint and amuses us by its behaviour. Some people value mink for the economic value of their fur, although they do not make good pets. We value cats rather than rats because they are pretty and can be tamed. But we appear to value people for some intrinsic worth just because they are people. We certainly don't value humans because they are rare. For example, we do not treat New Zealanders, because there are only 3 million of them, in preference to Americans who number 250 million. We do not favour Scotsmen rather than Englishmen because the former are about one tenth as common! To analyse the idea of value or worth further, we must ask several questions.

Does the value of a person change with age or abnormality?

Is a 20-year-old girl more valuable than an 80-year-old woman? If there has to be a choice between the two, say in the distribution of very limited food supplies, most would choose the young person and would justify it by saying the 80-year-old has had her life and has only a few more years left, whereas the 20-year-old has far more potential. The counter argument is that the old lady is far more helpless and unable to find food for herself. Different societies tend to put a different value on their elderly population. Many Eastern peoples have great reverence for old age and the elderly. In recent years in Britain, the elderly have lost a position of respect in society and are often put away into homes to be looked after and shamefully referred to in hospital as 'old crumble'. The question is, 'Does their worth alter because their bodies are crumbling?' We have to refer back, as we will have to again and again, to the basis of our value system. If mankind consists only of matter, and that matter is decaying, then, like an old rusty car, it loses its value. If however the human personality is transcendent, and more than just the chemicals and molecules that make up the body and brain, then the value of the personality remains, even though the body is crumbling. Despite that, we may still have to apply the criteria of 'potential' to difficult decision priorities.

When a person is severely handicapped she is still a human being and has the same intrinsic worth of a human being. The dignity of the elderly even if they are demented, lies in what they once were and now represent. Even the respect accorded to the dead body comes from what it represents in having housed a human spirit and personality. However, there are extreme cases at each end of life where the animate object before us seems less than fully human. For example, the anancephalic fetus, is alive in the womb but is incapable of more than a transitory independent existence, and the patient who is brain-dead, although heart and lungs are still working as long as the life support machine is switched on, may no longer be regarded as a person. Close to these extremes there is a group of difficult cases where the benefit of doubt about human worth must be given to the patient.

Does the value of a person change with the stage of development?

This is one of the two fundamental questions of the abortion debate (the other being the question of autonomy — *see* Chapter 8). So many thousands of words have been written on the subject and I will not repeat all the arguments here (*see* Further Reading). However, the views of different groups of people on the value of the embryo and fetus are so diametrically opposed, that I can see no possible common ground. Some women value their fetus in the same way that they value their gallbladder or appendix; if it is a nuisance and giving trouble, have it out! Yet most of these same women would not countenance infanticide; therefore, they make a fundamental distinction between the value of a dependent fetus and a free living baby. At the other extreme, there are those who claim that from the moment of conception the embryo has exactly the same value as a fully formed and independent human being. As usual, the views of most doctors, nurses and patients lie somewhere between these extremes. The difficulty is to identify a point at which there is a sudden change in the value of the developing embryo — when it develops a personality, when it has a soul. There appears to be a continuum of development, with no sudden changes. Many doctors take refuge in the concept of potential that was mentioned earlier. The value of a fetus, they argue, lies in the fact that it is a potential human person and that this potential increases with the age of the fetus, hence the recent efforts in Parliament to reduce the age at which abortions can be performed, because babies born at 24 weeks can now be kept alive independently of the mother and so 'the potential' has become 'actual'. Many of those (mainly Protestants) with a very conservative, but not absolutist, view on abortion, might argue that implantation and not conception, is the time when the potential starts; because a fertilized ovum has no potential, either in a test tube in the laboratory, or in the cavity of the uterus, until it has implanted. These people have no qualms about a contraceptive method that prevents implantation of the human conceptus (the IUCD), or about the destruction of embryos which are not required after *in vitro* fertilization with the husband's sperm, even though they might not countenance any form of abortion.

These questions are very important, for in Rex Gardner's words

> I who am due to perform an abortion tomorrow, must know whether I am to have a murder on my conscience.

When it comes to comparative values between mother and fetus, most practitioners, except staunch Roman Catholics, would have no doubt that the actual personality should be given preference over the potential life. Sometimes this is called *justifiable feticide*, a parallel being drawn with justifiable homicide, where one man is killed because he is threatening to kill another. What worried many people about the 1967 Abortion Act in Britain was that the value of the fetus was being weighed not only against the health and life of another human being (the mother), but against social factors and facilities as well. They urged that even potential people matter more than 'things'.

Does the value of a person change with social standing or function?

We must first ask: 'Of value to whom?' A theologian would stress that, in God's eyes, all men and women are equal but that, in the eyes of society, the Prime Minister may be of more value, at a particular time, than a road sweeper. If this is agreed (as it may or may not be) does this justify different priorities in medical treatment? To take the situation in China as another example: for some years, priority of medical care was given to those most useful to society, such as soldiers and farmers. In war time, in many countries, those soldiers who could be healed and returned to the battlefield were given priority over both those could not be restored, and also over the ordinary citizen. We know that this *does* happen; but the ethical question (as pointed out in Chapter 1) is *should* it happen? In an ideal world the answer would probably be 'No'; but if judgements have to be made, then those in leadership may be given priority, not because they are famous or wealthy or influential, but because they have responsibility for many other people. It is a matter of applying the right criteria in a particular situation. During World War II, Churchill was one of the few to be given some of the new scarce penicillin to treat his pneumonia. If there were objections to unfair privilege, it could also be argued that he was a privileged 'guinea pig'. [This is an unfortunate name because penicillin is toxic to guinea pigs!] But this principle of priority by function should operate only in special situations and not become ingrained in the ethical system. It is a proud boast of the British National Health Service that the surgeon who operates on the Queen also operates on the poorest of her subjects.

Does the value of a person change with different relationships?

One of the essences of being human is that loving relationships can be developed with other human beings. Often, when we are debating how much to strive to revive an elderly patient with many difficult problems, we hear the remark '. . . but she lives alone and has no relatives'. This is used as an argument for not trying too hard. We are assessing the value of the patient by her relationships or lack of them, and using that to try to assess the quality of her life and how much potential she has (*see* page 52).

To return to the abortion issue, many women do give a different value to the fetus after they have felt movements and therefore established a maternal relationship. Thus, 'quickening' has been proposed as a watershed after which abortion should not be performed. However, with modern ultrasound, mothers can see that their baby is, in fact, moving as early as 8 weeks of gestation, and this information does sometimes alter their attitude to termination of the pregnancy in the first trimester. A mother looking after three young children might justifiably be given priority in treatment over an older person with no responsibility or dependents because of a different function, rather than a different intrinsic worth. Does a person's value change when we dislike or disagree with them? There is a very important principle in this question, which is implicit in most of our codes of ethics and is explicit in the Declaration of Geneva:

> I will not permit considerations of religion, nationality, race, party politics or social standing to intervene between my duty and my patient.

In other words, there are no second class citizens when it comes to medical needs. This ethical principle is put to its greatest test in war time. It is a great credit to the British military and naval doctors and nurses that, in the Falklands War, they treated the Argentinian prisoners of war in just the same way as the British casualties. Indeed, they re-operated and saved the lives of a number who had been inadequately treated by their own medical officers.

But these recommendations are easier said than done. It is a credit to many Black and White doctors in South Africa that in spite of the règime, they are trying to build first-class care for the Black communities. But again we come back to the question 'Why should people of different races and backgrounds be treated alike?' For the Christian it only makes sense because of the value Christ demonstrated to all people of all races, and to the Humanist it makes sense because to do otherwise would demean the pre-eminent status of the human species. But for the true Marxist or Fascist, it is quite logical to treat different races differently.

The following is a useful aphorism to warn of the dangers of treating different patients in different ways based on personal opinions: 'Beware of the patient you dislike as well as the patient you like very much.' Your judgement can be biased by either and mistakes can be made.

This has been a brief sketch of the question of value, which is such an important ingredient in many ethical debates. The theory of value, known as axiology, has been debated for hundreds of years and is a subdivision within philosophy. For those who wish to pursue the arguments between the famous philosophers, suggested reading is given. For the rest, it is hoped that these questions have opened the eyes to the ways in which a sense of the value of a patient can alter medical practice. Respect for a patient is fundamental to the doctor/patient relationship and the respect we show, reflects what we think of the patient's worth.

References and Further Reading

See references under 'axiology' and 'value' in dictionaries of philosophy and ethics, and references to chapter 5.

Boyd K, Calaghan SJ and Shotter E (1986). *Life Before Birth: consensus in Medical Ethics*. SPCK, London.

Committee on the working of the abortion act (Lane report) (1974). HMSO, London.

Gardner RFR (1972). *Abortion: the Personal Dilemma*. The Paternoster Press, Exeter.

Review (1989). *Contemporary lessons from Nazi medicine*. Bulletin: **47**: 13–20. Institute of Medical Ethics.

8 Ethical component III: autonomy and consent

Autonomy is the third great theme in medical ethics and applies to both patients and their doctors. It means the freedom to determine one's own future without external restraints. It includes both the right to, and the capacity for, this self-determination and its implications in the ethical sphere were first given by Immanuel Kant.

The patient's autonomy

Medical practice throughout history has always been paternalistic from the days when the doctors were priests in ancient Egypt to the modern-day hospital consultant. The male domination of the medical profession has accentuated this paternalism. The patient is in a very vulnerable position because she is ill and dependent and does not possess the specialist knowledge and expertise of the doctor. The very jargon and language of medical practice creates a barrier between doctor and patient and puts the doctor on a pedestal. The sicker the patient, the more readily she accepts this 'vertical' relationship, partly because she has little choice and partly because a serious illness makes someone psychologically more dependent. The more powerful and technological that modern medicine becomes, the more the patient seems tied to a conveyor belt of investigation and treatment from which there is no escape. Many patients have been happy, in the past, to put implicit faith in the doctor because 'the doctor always knows best'. Some patients love to talk about 'doctor's orders', often to use them as an excuse for avoiding some unpleasant chore! But doctors should not give orders. In civilian practice, they are not in the relationship of a Commanding Officer to his men. It is the *patient's* illness, not the doctor's and the patient should be free to accept or reject the advice which she receives — or should she? Let us ask two subsidiary questions:

- Has the patient the right to autonomy?
- Is the patient capable of autonomy?

Has the patient a *right* to autonomy?

This question takes us back to the nature of a human being and his relationship to others in society. Do we believe in, and respect, the individual's personality as a unique individual? If so, why? Most societies recognize the right of their citizens to some degree of self-determination but this degree varies within different societies and at different times. There is less autonomy for the ordinary citizen in a strict Marxist règime than in a capitalist system, but in a time of war new restrictions are placed on citizens, even in a so-called 'free society'. Freedom is also restricted when that freedom puts other people at risk, and most societies use limitation of freedom in the form of imprisonment for those who have been judged to have abused that freedom. George Orwell's vision of 1984 is the ultimate picture of restriction of individual autonomy.

The question we must ask, then, is when a patient goes to a doctor to ask for advice and treatment, does she give up her autonomy — i.e., give up her right to influence the course of her treatment and make her own decisions about the future?

Is the patient *capable* of autonomy?

Whenever a certain elderly surgeon of my acquaintance was asked by a patient to explain what an operation involved, he used to reply 'It took me at least five years of intensive study to understand it, how do you expect me to explain it to you in five minutes' and then walked on to the next bed!

There are times when patients are not fit to exercise their own freedom of decision, such as when they are unconscious or severely mentally disturbed. In these cases, a close relative or friend takes temporary responsibility. Compulsory detention in a mental institution is used occasionally for the sake of protecting the patient and relatives, but the powers are strictly limited and temporary (new Mental Health Act). These situations are well-defined and rely, as do many others, on the social workers and doctors acting out of a sense of beneficence for the wellbeing of the patient. (But note that there may be a conflict, sometimes, between the benefit to the patients and the comfort of the relatives, who have to look after them.)

There are many common situations, where it is difficult for the patients to be truly informed. They have not, as that elderly surgeon realized, the background knowledge of anatomy, physiology or pathology to understand the details of medical procedures. But does this mean that they cannot understand sufficiently to make a responsible decision? As with all communication, the words do not matter as much as the meaning. This was brought home to me as a young surgeon when I was trying to explain to a rather deaf elderly woman that she needed an operation for intestinal obstruction. I was using words such as 'large bowel', 'obstructed' and 'fluid balance' and getting nowhere. Her son, who was a plumber, was standing at the bedside and could stand it no longer and blurted out 'You know Ma, the waste pipe's furred up. It needs to be chopped out and the other bits welded together.' She readily agreed to the operation!

It is medical language, more than anything else, that prevents the patient being fully informed. Fortunately, nowadays there is far more teaching in schools about human anatomy and physiology and far more understanding of disease. The key to giving the patients their autonomy is to respect them and not to talk down to them; it is vital to convey the facts in terms appropriate to that individual. Our respect for patients is determined by how much we value them as people. As a postscript, it is important to note that patients with medical knowledge often need as much careful explanation as their lay counterparts.

The philosophical theological question about the meaning of free will and how really free a person is to decide, is another fruitful area of study for those readers with a philosophical turn of mind. In philosophy, the debate is between Kant's thesis that all rational beings have the capacity to act in a consistently moral manner, irrespective of outside pressures, and the Determinism of Hobbes that every human action is causally conditioned. In theology, the debate is between the free will of the Armenians and the pre-destination of Calvin. For the sake of practical medical ethics, we must assume that the patient is able to make a rational decision, and that doctors must treat him in that way.

Consent to treatment

Lip-service is paid to the principle of informed consent in medical treatment and the patient's right not to have treatment without consent. Indeed, if a surgeon operates without consent, he lays himself open to a legal charge of assault. It is interesting, however, that written consent is required for surgical operations but not for certain drug treatments which are equally risky. The difference is that during an operation under an anaesthetic, a patient cannot decide that he does not wish to continue with the treatment, whereas when fully conscious it is assumed that he is in a position to say 'No' to a test, or refuse to take a drug. It is assumed that because a patient puts his arm out for a specimen of blood to be taken, he is consenting to that investigation. We shall see on page 126 that this implied consent has problems when it comes to testing for HIV. In practice, many patients do not even ask for information about their treatment; are they then really giving informed consent? Figure 8.1 is a standard consent form to operation, used in British National Health Service hospitals. In practice, some long word of Greek or Latin origin like 'Choledochoduodenostomy' is written in the space

G.906   OPERATION   CONSENT   FORMS

A. CONSENT BY PATIENT

I .... of .... hereby

consent to undergo the operation of .... the nature and purpose of which

have been explained to me by Dr./Mr. .... I also consent to such further or alternative operative measures as may be found to be necessary during the course of the operation, and to the
administration of a general, local or other anaesthetic for any of these purposes.

No assurance has been given to me that the operation will be performed by any particular surgeon.

Date .... Signed ....
                                                          (Patient)

I confirm that I have explained to the patient the nature and purpose of this operation.

Date .... Signed ....
                                                          (Physician/Surgeon)

Figure 8.1   A standard consent form to operation

at the top and patient is asked to sign at the bottom. Usually she will have been given a brief outline of the reason for the operation, where the incision will be and if there is a significant risk to life, but little more detail. The problem is that the doctor who gives, or does not give, that information is the one who signs he has done so! It might protect the patient's autonomy more if a third party, such as a nurse, signed that part, once she was satisfied that the patient understood. As it stands, should there be a disagreement about what information has been given, we only have the patient's word against the doctor's. In the USA, the consent form goes to the other extreme and every possible remote risk is itemized to cover the surgeon against litigation. As usual, some compromise between the two would be ideal, and with the increasing litigation in Britain, a rather more detailed consent form will probably be required. The present form, includes the phrase 'and other procedures which may be found necessary', so that if an unsuspected lesion is found, the patient does not have to be woken up in the middle of the operation to consent to a further procedure. This all depends on the surgeon obeying the two aims of medical care (*see* Chapter 6) of 1. only doing those things which will benefit the patient or are intended to benefit the patient, and 2. doing no intentional harm. It would only take one or two surgeons to abuse the remarkable trust that the patient puts in them, for the whole practice of consent to break down. Whether a patient is *capable* of fully informed consent will be discussed below, but there is no doubt that, at the present time in Britain, most patients are consenting to operations with very little information. This not only takes away their autonomy, but also puts an added burden on the surgeon, who has to make all the decisions.

When a group campaigns for 'rights', it is usually because some other group has not fulfilled its responsibilities. The recent increase in the number of 'patients' rights groups' and 'patients' associations' suggests that all is not well with the profession's approach to patient consent. Indeed, Carolyn Faulder in her challenging book *Whose Body Is It?* says that:

> far from being a matter of subsidiary interest, I maintain that informed consent is *the* ethical issue in medicine today and that unless we sort out our views and determine what we really mean when we talk about the patient's right to give informed consent, we are imperiling our ability to make wise and humane decisions about all the other bioethical problems now facing us'

Consent for research

This is an even more critical question and has two aspects depending on whether the subject is a patient or a healthy volunteer. This distinction is highlighted in the Declaration of Helsinki (p. 97).

Consent for research as a patient

This may involve various investigations and tests which may not affect the direct treatment of the disease but may help future patients. Often, however, the research involves a trial between two drugs or two forms of treatment. Sometimes one drug is inactive, a placebo, but this should only be used under two conditions:

1. When the disease is not serious and is self-limiting
2. Where there is strong subjective element to the condition so that a placebo effect is likely to be strong

Otherwise the comparison is made between an established treatment and a new treatment.

The key question is not only 'Should the patient be told that he is taking part in a drug trial?' to which the answer must usually be 'Yes'. But also 'At what stage should he be told?' In most trials, the two treatments are allocated randomly. Should the patient be told before randomization that the treatment will be decided by a toss of a coin or opening a sealed envelope, or should he be told after randomization that 'We have decided that such a treatment is the best one for you?' Patients may have difficulty in understanding the concepts and statistics behind randomization, but does that mean that they should have some of their autonomy taken away? If they are informed before randomization, some may refuse to take part and want to choose one treatment or the other, in the mistaken belief that either the new or the old must be better. Modern thinking is that the patient should be party to the decision about randomization and Carolyn Faulder argues strongly for this. Much depends on the relationship between the investigator and the patient, and Veitch suggests that the patient should be seen as a partner in the scientific enterprise rather than as a subject of research. This has much to recommend it. But written consent is still required for, as Paul Ramsey writes in his book *Patient as Person*, '. . . man's propensity to overreach a joint adventure, even in a good cause, makes consent necessary'. One of the weaknesses of the present system is that special ethical permission and consent is only required for formal trials and projects, not for a new treatment outside this framework. This problem is discussed further under Hospital Ethical Committees (p. 93).

Consent of healthy volunteers

This system is more clear cut. Autonomy dictates that the subjects are free to participate or not as they wish, because they do not *need* any of the investigations or the treatment. However, this autonomy may be eroded in two ways:

1. By 'moral' pressure. This is why the Declaration of Helsinki recommends that subjects who are in a direct subordinate relationship with the investigator should not be used. It is very difficult for a medical student to refuse the Professor's request to volunteer for a study if the Professor adds '. . . and my house job comes up in six months' time!'

2. By financial pressure. Payment of volunteers has become accepted practice but until recently was frowned upon by the Research Councils because of the risk that financial incentives might be used to limit the subject's freedom. The compromise position is that the payment is appropriate to the time and trouble involved in research and possible loss of wages during the study.

The use of prisoners with the inducement of remission that has been used in the USA has not been countenanced in Britain, for the same reasons. Although it could be argued that a prisoner's autonomy has already been taken away and this would speed up the time when he gets it back!

The right to accurate information

This will be discussed more in the next chapter but is, again, a relevant question. Carolyn Faulder has also pointed out that autonomy includes the right *not* to have the information if you do not want it — not have it 'forced down your throat'.

Limitation of rights

Although we may all be agreed that patient autonomy is justified and should be safeguarded and protected, there are some areas where the patient's right to freedom may have to be limited. These are to be considered under several headings.

When the patient's autonomy could affect others

The classical example of this is the compulsory isolation or restriction of a patient with an infective disease. In Britain this is not as important as it was, when diseases such as smallpox, tuberculosis and poliomyelitis were rife, but the State had the power to compel isolation and treatment for the sake of others. State power can be dangerous and this ability to restrict the patient's freedom should only be sanctioned under four conditions:

1. Other avenues of control have been exhausted or are inappropriate
2. The risk of spread is very high and the disease serious
3. Only those who are affecting others must be restricted
4. It is done by the proper authorities, openly.

Smallpox came under these categories but paratyphoid does not, although the patient is banned from working with food and so, temporarily, may lose employment.

A second example is inherent in the abortion debate. The right of autonomy is summed up in the statement 'it is the women's right to decide'. This is only valid if the fetus is not considered to be another person relevant to the discussion. Autonomy might have to be restricted if the life of a third party is at risk.

A third example is the status of Jehovah's Witnesses. A mentally sound adult is perfectly entitled to put stipulations on his treatment, such as not wanting a blood transfusion, but when this puts a child's life at risk, British law puts a limit on the freedom of one person to decide about another: the child is either made a ward of court or, if time is too short, the doctor may proceed with the transfusion having obtained written agreement of a colleague supporting his opinion that transfusion is necessary (BMA Handbook).

Have patients the right to harm themselves?

This question includes the right to refuse treatment that could be life-saving. If patients have the right to accept treatment, they must also have the right to refuse it, but it is the doctor's responsibility to make sure they have all the information so that they know the consequences of their refusal. It is interesting that most doctors give far more honest information to a patient refusing treatment than to one accepting it! Has the patient the right to harm himself by continuing to smoke or drink excessive alcohol and then expect medical treatment for the consequences? Many surgeons refuse to operate on a patient with arterial disease unless he stops smoking because any benefit would be very shortlived. By so doing, they accept the patient's right to harm himself if he wishes, but not his right to insist on treatment for the consequences. Some patients consider it as an intrusion on their freedom for the doctor to advise them to change their lifestyles: 'I can do what I like and it is up to the National Health Service to treat me. After all I pay my stamps!' is a caricature of this view. It is interesting, and illogical, that advice on eating, drinking or smoking is permissible whereas advice on sexual behaviour to avoid venereal disease and unwanted pregnancy is considered 'judgemental.'

The compulsory wearing of car seat-belts is now law in Britain, but only after a number of attempts to get the legislation through Parliament. At one time there was a strong argument that this was an infringement of the individual's right to risk injury or kill himself, if he wished. It was claimed that if an individual did not wear a seat-belt, it would not harm others (but only give more work to the Health Service!). The same people who objected to compulsory seat-belts in cars would happily wear one in an aeroplane, although, there, it is far less likely to prevent injury. Such compulsory protective legislation is common in factories and the safety of factory workers in Britain has been greatly enhanced by compulsory regulations. Public Health measures such as the prevention of toxic emissions from factories are very effective if they do not depend on an individual's will-power. However, solving the huge public health problems of smoking, alcohol abuse and sexually transmitted diseases depends on education and persuasion and this has largely failed, because of the weakness of human nature.

A final example is suicide. The present law in Britain is that someone is not charged for attempted suicide but the person who assists him may be charged. The Law, therefore, recognizes a person's right to take his own life but not his right to involve a third party in the killing, because the dividing line between assisting suicide and murder is very fine. Recently, an attempt has been made, which failed, to alter this law and legalize assisting suicide as a way of opening the door to voluntary euthanasia. To answer the question whether suicide or aiding suicide is wrong or not, we must return to the fundamentally different views of human nature outlined in Chapter 5. If death is the extinction of the personality and I am answerable to no one but myself — if 'I am the captain of my fate, I am the master of my soul' — then suicide is a logical way of ending my life, providing it does not upset friends and relatives. If, however, to aid a person's suicide might be to plunge him into hell, that is a very different matter; if I am answerable to God and will have to explain my actions when I meet him, I need to think twice.

The doctor has a responsibility to treat someone who has attempted suicide by poisoning because it is assumed that the 'balance of the patient's mind was disturbed' in the absence of any evidence to the contrary. However, in the case of a hunger strike in prison, where there is plenty of time to check that the patient is of sound mind and understands what he is doing, the doctor is not obliged to 'force-feed'. This is the advice of the *BMA Handbook of Medical Ethics* and is a good example for a discussion on autonomy.

The doctor's autonomy

If we are to respect the patient's autonomy, what about the *doctor's* freedom? Clinical freedom has been the doctor's watchword for years and has meant that nothing must intervene between him and his patient. It has sometimes been used as a cloak for less than ideal medical ethics. One consultant in the NHS might claim that he had the right to treat all his patients with the newest expensive drug, even if it meant that other areas of care would be short of money. Does clinical freedom include the right to choose the conditions and place of work as well as the right to make a particular clinical decision about a patient? Clinical freedom, as an unalterable right, is wearing a bit thin under the conditions of twentieth century practice. Rights also involve responsibilities — responsibilities in the use of scarce resources, and there are several areas where doctors' rights and freedoms should be questioned.

Moral pressure from authorities

There is a distinction between authorities exerting a justified control over a doctor's activities and bringing pressure to bear on his moral and ethical position. For example, to safeguard a doctor's freedom, it was essential that the 1967 Abortion Law had a conscience clause so that a doctor or nurse with a conscientious objection to abortion could not be forced to participate. Although this clause may have been effective for those already in post at the time of the Act, it has not always been honoured in appointments committees for gynaecological and anaesthetic posts. There has, in addition, been a number of recent cases where Health Authorities have misused their powers to suspend a doctor from practice: whereas these powers were designed to protect patients from a sick or dangerous doctor, they have been used to suspend doctors — sometimes for years — while alleged irregularities of finances were being investigated which had no bearing on the safety or standards of patient care.

The right of doctors to act in the best interests of their patients independently of outside pressure is embodied in the Declaration of Geneva:

> . . . even under *threat* I will not use my medical knowledge contrary to the laws of humanity.

The Declaration of Tokyo (1975) giving guidelines for doctors in relationship to torture and other inhumane and degrading treatments, states:

> . . . a doctor must have complete clinical independence in deciding upon the care of a person for whom he or she is medically responsible (*see* page 101).

Clinical freedom is a freedom to do good, and like any freedom carries responsibilities which must not be abused.

Pressure from patients

Respect for the doctor/patient relationship must be mutual. In an abortion decision, has the doctor the right to force her moral views on the patient? By the same token, has the patient the right to force her moral views on the doctor? If the doctor is conscientiously opposed to abortion on moral grounds, she must say so openly and should not be forced to concede to a patient's request. A patient should have the freedom to visit another practitioner. In this way, both doctor and patient keep their autonomy, their respect for each other and their consciences clear. This is not to say that doctors should never discuss the pros and cons with the patient, but in the discussion, they must make it clear which are moral and which are medical criteria.

Often the patients' attempts at persuasion are on a very much more mundane level, such as requesting a certain treatment. They may demand antibiotics for a cold, or 'the tablets that my friend was given.' If the doctor does not think the treatment is justified, she might refuse, pointing out the drug is not necessary and could have side-effects. Is this violating the patient's freedom? Surely the patient's right is to a sound medical opinion, not necessarily to a particular drug.

Second opinions

Many doctors feel very threatened when a patient asks for a second opinion, but this should not be construed as undermining their autonomy. All doctors must recognize they are sometimes wrong and often need further advice from colleagues. For a patient to be able to ask for a second opinion, under special circumstances, is an important freedom which some highly socialized healthcare systems have taken away.

The doctor must be free *not* to break the law!

One of the most worrying aspects of the first guidelines emerging after the Gillick case (see Chapter 13) about giving contraception to under-16-year-olds without telling their parents, was that doctors were instructed that, if they complied with the law and *did* tell the parents, they could be disciplined. In other words, the principle of confidentiality was held to supercede the law. This recommendation has now been altered, so that the doctor is free to prescribe, under special circumstances, if he considers it in the best interest of his patient *not* to tell her parents. In other words, if he decides to break the law for a very good reason, he may be protected. On the other hand, a psychiatrist may lay himself open to being held in contempt of court if he decides to refuse to break the confidences of a patient who is under trial. He is in a very difficult position but he has the freedom either to tell or not to tell and to take the consequences. Is this any different from the pressure of the authorities referred to above?

In summary, the doctor should have clinical freedom to do what he thinks is in the best interest of his patient. Patients and doctors should respect each other's freedoms within the doctor/patient relationship. Pressures on this autonomy come from many quarters and cause some of the most important arguments in medicine today.

References and Further Reading

British Medical Association (1981). *The Handbook of Medical Ethics*.
Faulder C (1985). Whose Body is it? In *The Troubling Issue of Informed Consent*. Virago, London.

Hoffenberg R (1987). *Clinical Freedom.* The Nuffield Provincial Hospital Trust, London.

Kant I (1949). *The Critique of Practical Reason,* (ed and trans) Jeevis White. University of Chicago Press, Chicago.

Kant I (1964). *The Metaphysics of Morals,* (trans) Mary Gregor. Harper and Row, New York.

Ramsay P (1976). *Patient as Person.* Yale University Press, New Haven, Connecticut and London.

Veatch RM (1987). *The Patient as Partner.* Indiana University Press, Indianappolis.

9 Ethical component IV: truth and integrity

How extraordinary that a book on medical ethics should have a section on truth! Surely it is self-evident that doctors tell the truth? After all, they are well-educated people! Ethics it might be argued should be concerned with the more important matters such as '*in vitro*' fertilization and genetic engineering. Perhaps these were your thoughts on seeing the chapter heading. It is interesting how people love to discuss the great unsolvable problems, but ignore the way that ethical principles are broken every day in the course of the simple doctor/patient interaction. The important problem is that, in the past, doctors have been fairly consistent liars, if not in their private lives, certainly in their medical practice. Perhaps 'deceivers' would be a better word than 'liars' because they have usually given the impression that the diagnosis was not what it actually was, without necessarily saying so outright. Often in the past, consultants have put their nursing and social worker colleagues in a very difficult position by this policy of hiding the diagnosis of cancer from a patient. I have even known a consultant request the pathology department to type out a false pathology report to try to convince the patient that he did not have cancer, when he did! This policy is all the more extraordinary when one considers the average doctor's reaction when the patient lies to *him*. When he finds out he might exclaim 'How can I possibly help you if you do not tell me the truth?' How did this situation arise, for it was not always so? When did lying doctors become 'respectable'? In Victorian times, judging by the novels, patients were regularly told they were dying and how long they had to live. That was in the days when very little could be done to avert the course of the disease. Now we have a whole range of potent therapies, yet we have turned, as a profession, to being more deceptive, less able to deal with the truth.

This situation probably arose in the 1930s and '40s when accurate diagnosis outstripped effective treatment and the doctor's dilemma became acute. An individual doctor's policy can often be traced back to one unfortunate experience when a patient reacted 'very adversely' to the bad news. The doctor then vowed never to tell a patient the full truth again. However, it is very unwise to base a policy on one unfortunate experience, whether in surgery or ethics. Nowadays there is a welcome return to more honest dealings with patients, although there may be a danger of over-swing to an insensitive truth-telling by some. In the USA, doctors have been far more open with their patients, perhaps due to the influence of litigation (see Chapter 13).

Why tell the truth?

In the same way that we had to ask, in Chapter 7, why we value human beings, we must ask, here, why we should tell the truth to patients. No question exposes our basic philosophies more starkly. A Christian, who claims to follow Christ who said 'I am the truth', finds it difficult to tell a lie or plan to deceive his fellow man. However, a utilitarian, who justifies his actions only by their results, might consider lying good, if it gives the patient peace of mind. Often such people look only at the short-term effect. Later, if the patient finds he has been deceived, or a relative becomes ill himself and wonders whether he has been told the truth or not, the long-term results may not be so good. It is far better that the patient should be given the opportunity to restore strained relationships and prepare for death (and the world to come) while there is still time and he is still alert. So there are reasons of principle to tell the truth to patients, but there are also two other justifications: namely, that of respect for the patient and that of the patient's autonomy, which we have discussed above. The patient cannot make decisions affecting her own illness and treatment if she does not know her diagnosis and her prognosis.

What is the truth?

We do not always know the truth about an illness, and when we think we do, we can sometimes be wrong. It is most unwise to tell patients facts until we are sure. Integrity also demands that we admit when we do not know what is wrong. To pretend is to deceive, and the doctor's fear that patients will no longer respect one, who honestly says he does not know, is usually unfounded. The following cautionary tale illustrates some of the problems of telling patients what is wrong with them:

> A patient from overseas was visiting the USA for a conference and developed obstructive jaundice. He was operated on and found to have a lump in his pancreas, which was thought to be a cancer

obstructing his bile duct, and an operation to by-pass it was performed. Unusually, for the USA, he was told there was no cancer but his wife was told the true diagnosis. He could not understand why his wife was so sad. I was asked to see him 18 months later, when he was still jaundiced. I re-operated and found that the cause of his jaundice was a gallstone which was also partly blocking the by-pass and the 'lump' in his pancreas was a benign cyst. I told him and his wife the good news and his wife was, of course, overjoyed. The original surgeon had thought he was telling the patient a lie and his wife the truth, when in fact it was the other way round!

There is a fundamental difference between lying and making an unintentional mistake, as Richard Cabot has pointed out in his classic treatise, 'Honesty':

> There is no such thing as an unintended lie. Everyone of us makes unintended mistakes about *facts* every day.

There is a difference between *veracity* and *infallibility*. He goes on to say that:

> the greatest medical liars that I have known have been duffers at diagnosis, with little or nothing clear in their own minds as to what ails the patient. It is easy for them to tell him a pleasing lie.

Possible exceptions to the principle of truth-telling will be discussed on page 73) and an analysis of what to tell the patients with cancer in Chapter 14. Sissela Bok's first-class book *Lying* is well worth studying as she discusses the problem in relationship to political as well as medical life.

Integrity: it involves far more than just telling the truth

It includes such areas as honesty in financial matters, and in research, where the temptation to take credit directly, or by implication, for research performed by others is particularly strong. The book *Betrayers of the Truth* by William Broad and Nicholas Wade is a devastating exposé of the lack of integrity in research throughout the ages. Even Mendel is accused of 'cooking' the figures for his famous genetic experiments with sweet peas! The question of integrity is one of the important ethical issues in research today with the tremendous pressure to publish large numbers of papers for one's *Curriculum Vitae* or future research grants.

Promise-keeping: keeping faith with the patient

From the patient's point of view, it is very important that doctors and nurses are reliable and keep their promises. If they fail to keep small promises such as 'I will come back and see you again tomorrow' how can the patient trust them over much larger matters: 'I will take your appendix out at the same time as your ovarian cyst.' Ill patients have many unjustified anxieties, but confidence in the doctor is not primarily built up by his claims to do marvellous things, but rather in his being utterly reliable and not two-faced or capricious. This is beginning to look like a tall order, which allows only paragons of virtue to apply for medicine! By the very nature of the health professions, and the responsibility and power that they wield, integrity must be high on the list of required qualities. There are plenty of temptations in the opposite direction and plenty of opportunities, both in care of patients and medical research, to bend the rules. (How many doctors do, actually, inspect the body before signing a cremation form, for which they are paid a significant fee?)

One of the best examples to illustrate this and some of the other ethical components we have discussed so far, is the varying attitudes of surgeons to operations on Jehovah's Witnesses. Jehovah's Witnesses, from deeply held religious convictions, do not allow themselves to be given blood transfusions. They believe that if they have a transfusion they are condemned eternally, so they would rather die quickly and preserve their spiritual life than survive physically and lose eternal life. The doctor may admire their sense of priorities but disagree with their action and their interpretation of a difficult verse in the Old Testament, but that is not relevant to this illustration. When a surgeon is asked to operate on a Jehovah's Witness he has three choices:

1. To refuse to operate under the restriction of 'no transfusions'
2. To agree to operate, while promising not to transfuse blood even if there is severe haemorrhage
3. To agree to operate on the patient's terms, but put up a blood transfusion under the anaesthetic if it is needed, without the patient knowing, and taking it down again before he wakes up.

The first of these actions preserves the doctor's autonomy and integrity but not the patient's because he does not receive treatment under the conditions he desires. The second preserves the patient's autonomy but not the doctor's: the doctor's freedom is restricted by the patient's demands, but his integrity is preserved. Legally, there is no problem provided the patient signs a special consent form. The third course of action preserves neither the patient's autonomy nor the doctor's integrity. The doctor has not kept his promise and, if discovered (because he had not changed the giving set and the blood could be seen in the drip chamber!) loses all trust and respect from the patient in the future. Even if he is not discovered, he has acted deceitfully. If he is a deontologist (*see* p. 5) he will be wrong, but if he is a teleologist, he may well congratulate himself for having pulled off the deception 'in the patient's best interest'.

Another time when keeping faith with the patient is very important, and which is linked with truth-telling, is the response to a patient who, before operation, asks a straight question 'Will you please tell me if you find evidence of cancer?' Having agreed to this request, the doctor must keep his promise. How much to tell the patient if she has *not* asked is another question. But here is a direct agreement and a promise made, which must be kept, even if the findings are unexpected and the news unpleasant.

A third classical example is an epileptic patient who refuses to tell the Motor Licensing Authority about his condition. How can the doctor keep faith with him? She must advise him very strongly to give the information, but if that fails she might have to warn him that it is her duty to tell the authorities for the sake of pedestrians and other road users. She keeps faith with him by telling him what she is going to do, rather than 'sneaking' behind his back. A very similar situation arises when a patient is a known typhoid carrier and continues to work in a restaurant. In the complicated world of clinical medicine, the wise doctor is careful about the promises that he makes!

Are there exceptions to truth-telling?

Many of the most ardent supporters of truth admit that there are a few occasions where a lie or half-truth is justified. The classical example discussed years ago by Samuel Johnson, is when a murderer asks you which way a potential victim has gone. It is argued that it is justified to give the murderer false information, to save the man's life and to avert a serious crime. Kant, on the other hand, argued that, even when you do tell the murderer the truth, you are not responsible for the crime itself; the murderer still has to commit it (see discussion by Sissela Bok in *Lying*, page 40).

Some doctors have drawn a parallel between this situation, which might justify a lie, and the clinical problems when the patient threatens that he will commit suicide if he finds out he has cancer. By telling him a lie, that he does not have cancer, you might be saving his life, temporarily. In both illustrations there is variable doubt whether the murder or suicide will, in fact, be committed but in the first case, the victim has no autonomy (freedom) in relation to his death, whereas the second victim still has autonomy of action. The principles and implications of telling patients they have cancer will be discussed more fully in Chapter 14.

Confidentiality

In order for a doctor to help a patient, he has to be given confidential facts that the patient does not wish to be passed to a third person. The sensitivity of these facts varies considerably between different branches of medicine, from psychiatry, gynaecology and genitourinary medicine on the one hand to orthopaedics and ENT on the other. Patients do not usually mind others knowing that they have a sore throat or a fractured wrist, but are not so keen for their sexual activities to be made public. So, patients, quite naturally, are sensitive about medical details that the doctor might not suspect and the patients would argue that they, and not the doctor, should decide what should be told. Confidentiality has been a part of a medical ethical code throughout the ages. The Hippocratic Oath says nothing about telling the truth to the patient, but has a strong clause on confidentiality:

> whatever in connection with my professional practice, or not in connection with it, I see or hear in the life of men which ought not to be spoken of abroad, I will not divulge as reckoning that all such be kept secret.'

The Declaration of Geneva states:

> I will respect the secrets which have been confided in me, even after the patient has died.

The Hippocratic Oath includes items that the doctor has learnt *outside* his professional relationships. This is an interesting area for discussion, but it must be remembered that a doctor is also a citizen and he has a duty to report to the police any events he has witnessed or observed which *any other citizen* could have observed. That is very different from letting the police know details that a patient has told him in the course of professional consultation or things he has observed because he visited a house at the patient's request. The Declaration of Geneva has added '. . . even after the patient has died' and this presents a problem for historians. There was considerable debate at the end of the 1960s when Winston Churchill's doctor published medical details about him after his death. Certainly, hospital records must still be stored confidentially or destroyed after a patient has died.

Why is confidentiality important?

There are at least three reasons, two of principle and one of consequence.

The patient's autonomy

Facts and details belong to the patient. They have been given to the doctor for a certain purpose, so that an illness can be treated and the patient given advice, and on certain understandings — that the doctor will not divulge them. It has always seemed extraordinary to me that hospital notes are often labelled 'Not to be handled by the patient' when they should read 'Not to be handled by anybody else without the patient's permission'!

The doctor's integrity

He has made certain implicit undertakings to the patient about what he will do with the information and breaks his promise if he divulges it.

The consequences for the future relationship

If confidences *are* broken, patients in the future will not tell the doctor vital information which could lead to a misdiagnosis or wrong treatment.

Many readers may think that this is all obvious, is agreed by everyone and is not really a problem. Unfortunately, patients' confidences are broken every day in all sorts of ways and while Ethical Committees are debating the minutiae of research projects, patients' secrets are being broadcast far and wide. I have, therefore, reviewed three problem areas related to confidentiality: firstly, *breaches* of confidentiality, secondly, *safeguards* of confidentiality, and thirdly, *exceptions* to confidentiality.

Breaches of confidentiality

Since this section already sounds like a three-point sermon, it will be appropriate to classify these failures in the same way as the Prayer Book — into *negligence*, *weakness* and our *own deliberate fault*!

Negligence

Most breaches of confidentiality, certainly in hospital practice, occur through carelessness, such as gossiping in the lifts or on the bus on the way home. It is easy to leave notes open on the desk to be read by all and sundry. It is quite appropriate that patient's problems should be discussed in case conferences, which involve many different types of health workers, all with the patient's best interest at heart, but some details need not be aired in public and it is very easy for information to be given unintentionally to people who are not bound by professional ethics (the British Association of Social Workers Ethical Code is not supported by the same sanctions as those exercised by the General Medical Council or the Council for Professions Allied to Medicine).

In September 1988, the Department of Health issued guidelines to safeguard identifiable personal information held in the records of local authorities for the purpose of their social services functions. Receptionists and secretaries have a particular responsibility. Although it does not always have the desired effect, the typing of 'confidential' or 'personal' on the envelope at least absolves the secretary of responsibility if it is opened by another person. The following true illustration previously published (Bliss and Johnson, 1975) is a poignant reminder.

> Some years ago, a patient with varicose veins was admitted for operation. Among routine blood tests performed was a test for syphilis. The patient was in the ward only a few days and a positive result came back after he had gone home. The doctor who received the result wrote to him explaining that a test for syphilis had proved to be positive and he was enclosing an appointment for the VD Clinic. The letter came through the door at a time when the patient was busy and, seeing it was from the hospital, he asked his daughter to open it and to read it out — with its embarrassing revelation. When the patient saw the venereologist, another test proved that the finding was a false positive and there was no evidence that the patient had syphilis at all! Fortunately, the patient and his family took it all in good part and recognized that the doctor had been trying to do his best.

General practitioners' receptionists and nurses in a small community are particularly vulnerable to breaking confidences, because they often know their patients at a personal level and may know their friends and neighbours as well. It is so easy to reply without thinking, to the innocent question 'How is Mrs Wilson?' by giving more detail than is necessary. In hospital, it is important not to put the diagnoses on any operating or admission list that will be displayed on a notice board.

Weakness

Nurses in hospital have a particular problem when answering telephone calls which are usually genuine, but occasionally are not. Nurses are taught to give only the minimal details in answer to enquiries over the telephone unless they are quite sure of the identity of the caller. That is why their answers often seem so unhelpful and non-committal. Sadly, both the press and employers sometimes pose as anxious relatives and sometimes a relative is also an employer!

The media

Unfortunately, the media as a whole are not interested in confidentiality and many journalists have no ethical code. The editors' prime aim is to sell their newspapers and controversy and half-truths are their means. Although some doctors have told half-truths for the sake of their patients, journalists tell half-truths for the sake of their pockets. This is a generalization, of course, and there are notable exceptions, but it cannot be said of journalists as a whole that their overriding concern is for the good of the patient. Most television programmes are devised primarily to entertain and secondarily to inform. Maximum controversy gives the best entertainment. The other great problem with the media is that they do not understand that truth consists of the balance of facts, not just one statement. They think that by quoting one part of a sentence accurately they are conveying the truth, whereas leaving out the qualifying clause at the beginning of the sentence, completely alters its sense. The deception is not always intentional, but it can be very destructive. Accurate reporting is often spoiled by the caption writers who were not at the original interview and who completely distort the report, by highlighting one small part. All health workers must be very careful about speaking to the press about patients. The best rule is to speak to the person only through the press officer in a hospital, who will make a prepared statement usually cleared with the patient or relatives. A good journalist will allow his report to be checked for accuracy by the doctor or administrator concerned.

Non-professional staff in hospital

It is easy for porters, electricians, plumbers and other essential hospital staff, not directly involved in the care of patients, to have access to notes, either when transporting the patient or when carrying out repairs in the filing room. I have seen an electrician looking at notes as a welcome break from replacing strip lighting!

Intentionally

Unfortunately, pressure in the form of financial inducements is sometimes placed on healthcare workers to reveal confidential details. Sometimes these details are spread from a motive of malicious gossip. All contracts for health workers, who do not have their own professional ethic, should contain a confidentiality clause which, if broken intentionally, can be the means of disciplinary action.

Safeguards of confidentiality

A number of these have been mentioned in the previous section. The great safeguard is to divulge no information without the patient's written permission. This particularly applies to reports to solicitors and employers. The passing of hospital or general practice notes to a third party must only be done with permission. Technically the notes belong to the administrators of the hospital but they normally check with the consultant in charge of the patient. Courts of law now have the power to subpoena the hospital notes. Computer-held records are subject to the Data Protection Act (1984) and patients may have access to any records held on computer.

Anonymity

Details about patients are used widely for health statistics and research. This is perfectly permissible provided that the information is anonymous. The health statisticians and health planners do not need to know that Mr MacDonald has arthritis but they do need to know that a man of 70, living alone, has arthritis. When publishing case histories or reports, the patient's name is omitted and any clinical photograph made unrecognizable. The following is a good general rule where health workers are discussing their work, at home or socially:

- If you mention the condition, do not mention the patient's name
- If you mention the patient's name, do not mention the condition
- Only tell friends that a patient is ill if they have already discovered it from another source

Relatives

One of the extraordinary ethical inconsistencies of modern medical practice is that if a fully rational patient has cancer, it is common practice to tell the relatives first and the patient later, or not at all. If a patient has a sexually transmissible disease or is HIV-positive, no one would dream of telling the relatives first. Consistency is an important aspect of ethical thinking. How has this inconsistency arisen? It comes, no doubt, from the laudable desire to protect the patient from unpleasant news but the relatives' reactions are frequently: 'He must not know! You won't tell him, will you?' Indeed, well meaning relatives must bear a large responsibility for the present state of affairs of not telling patients about their disease. Surely both the principle of autonomy and that of confidentiality demand that the patient is told something first and at least she *knows* that the doctor is talking to her relatives. She might wish one relative to be told, but not another. Not all family relationships are equally harmonious.

Patients' access to their own notes

A number of general practices are adopting the policy of allowing patients to see their own notes and the letters and reports from hospitals. Some even leave the practice notes in the patient's possession permanently, which makes life much simpler during night calls and when a deputizing service is on call. This policy would seem to be justified by autonomy and confidentiality, the patient being the guardian of his own confidences. However, the British Medical Association is strongly opposed to any rule that allows patients to be able to see their own notes, arguing that these are the doctor's records of the patient's illness. As usual, there is a middle road, but unless more information is regularly given to patients there will be increasing demands for access. On the other hand, hospital doctors may modify or abbreviate their reports if they know the letter will be read by the patient.

Exceptions to confidentiality

In the previous section we mentioned a possible exception to truth-telling. Are there any exceptions to the principle of confidentiality? Several have already been mentioned but they can be summarized as follows:

1. When the patient gives consent
2. When the doctor has an overriding duty to society
3. When the information is required by due legal process, e.g., notification of infectious diseases, evidence to the courts
4. When patients found to have a genetically related disease or to be a carrier of an abnormal gene and other members of the family may also need to be told that they could be carriers.

In regard to the compulsory disclosure of medical records in case of personal injury or death, the Administration of Justice Act 1970, Section 31, reads as follows:

On the application in accordance with rules of Court of a person who appears to the High Court likely to be a party to subsequent proceedings in that Court in which a claim in respect of personal injuries to a person or in respect of a person's death is likely to be made, the High Court shall in certain circumstances, as may be specified in the rules, have power to order a person who appears to the Court to be likely to be a party to proceedings and is likely to have or to have had in his possession, custody or power any documents which are relevant to an issue arising or likely to arise out of that claim (a) to disclose where these documents are in his possession, custody or power; and (b) to produce to the applicant such of these documents as are in his possession, custody or power.

However, more often the doctor is caught off his guard when a policeman asks for details in the hospital accident and emergency department. A police surgeon examining a patient on behalf of the police is in a special non-therapeutic role and the patient has the right to refuse to be examined or to provide specimens for forensic examination. There is a risk that if police are given details about a patient under treatment, that right of refusal will be lost. This is different from a proper police statement as part of the investigation of an accident or crime. The doctor should tell the police, however, whether or not a patient is fit to be seen and questioned.

It will be seen from this account how easily confidentiality can be broken and it is encumbent on all health workers to safeguard the patients' secrets by all possible means.

References and Further Reading

Bliss BP and Johnson AG (1975). *Aims and Motives in Clinical Medicine*. Pitman Medical, London.
Bok S (1980). *Lying*. Quartet Books, London.
Broad W and Wade N (1983). *Betrayers of the Truth*. Century Publishing, London.
Cabot RD (1938). *Honesty*. McMillan, New York.

10 Absolutes:
through-ways only

Implicit in the concept of pathways is that the traveller reaches junctions on the way, where he has to decide which way to go. But some fellow explorers appear to find the journey very simple and seem not to have to make difficult decisions on the way. These people are of two types: those who have absolute rigid ethical principles from which there are no deviations and no extenuating circumstances, and, secondly, those who have no ethical principles and so can wander where they like and just take whichever path they feel moved to join at the time (the subjective existentialist of Chapter 5). Life is much more easy for these two groups than for most people who are standing at the road junction, scratching their heads, wondering which way to turn (Fig. 1.1). The teleologist tries to see in the distance where each path leads (i.e., the result of his decision) and the deontologist looks back to see the direction she has come (takes a compass-bearing to make sure the path is in line with her principles), and only deviates from its direction if there is a clear signpost elsewhere. Let us look at some ethical principles that could be considered absolutes.

The sanctity of human life

This is one of the most familiar ethical phrases, especially in religious circles. Some religions (e.g. Buddhists) apply it to all types of life, as did Albert Schweitzer, the famous missionary in Africa. What does it mean? Does it mean that human physical life is inviolable, never to be taken under any circumstances? Or does it mean that human life should be held in a unique esteem as compared with other forms of life? It must be very difficult to practise modern medicine if the life of a mosquito, that is carrying malaria, or a rat, that is carrying the plague, is given the same respect as human life. The relationship of 'man' to the rest of creation is fundamental to this discussion (see Chapter 7 and Chapter 16).

The Declaration of Geneva, as we have seen, uses the words 'utmost respect for human life'. Utmost seems to imply that nothing can be more important — except, perhaps, another human life. So this might include the situation where a policeman shot a man who was just about to kill another (justifiable homicide) or the termination of a fetus that was threatening the life of a mother (justifiable feticide). Those who do not countenance abortion on any grounds argue that the fetus needs special protection because it is innocent, dependent and cannot speak for itself. As we have already pointed out, the divergence of views will never be resolved. Is it possible to hold a very high view of human life but still allow for the occasional exception? It is, provided the exceptions are clearly defined and still regarded as exceptions to a principle, rather than the norm. This is difficult to maintain in practice. 'The lesser of two evils' concept will be discussed in the next chapter but the exception can prove the rule rather than invalidate it. As Professor Dunstan (qv) points out, the Judaeo–Christian root from which the term 'sanctity' is derived (holy or set apart) also allowed judicial killing, and in Jewish and Christian thinking, life included the whole personality not just the physical body. This is particularly relevant to the question of brain death, which is one of the ethical areas about which there is a wide measure of agreement. Doctors and the general public have all accepted the concept that with no detectable brain function, the personality has gone, and *the patient as a person is dead*, although the heart may be beating and the lungs artificially ventilated. The Declaration of Sydney (p. 95) provides the widely accepted criteria and safeguards. A slightly irreverent story brings home this point:

> A patient died and went to heaven, and as he passed the entrance door he was chuckling with laughter. St Peter asked him why he was so amused. 'Can't you see' he replied, 'they still have my body on a life support machine down there!'

Truth-telling

This has been discussed in the last chapter but is a good example. A 'through-way policy' could be always to tell the patient 'the truth, the whole truth, and nothing but the truth', not even holding back any detail. Most people do not do this in everyday relationships. They do not tell a friend exactly what they think about him or her, but 'they temper justice with mercy'. Compassion is a temporizing force to the amount of truth we tell. This is very different from making lies the norm. Surprising though it may seem, in the past, some doctors had the absolute policy that patients with cancer should *never* be told the truth!

Prolonging life at all costs

This is a possible absolute that was mentioned in Chapter 6. The justification for this lies in a concept of life that is physical and that is judged in terms of quantity rather than quality. It is important to point out here a common source of confusion. There are four actions, with different ethical implications, when we are considering the termination of life:

1. Turning off the respirator when a patient is judged to be brain-dead, which to the great majority is now no longer an ethical problem.

2. Deciding not to resuscitate a patient with terminal disease whose heart has stopped. This would be prolonging death rather than life. Cardiac arrest is the normal final end to physical life.

3. Giving pain-killers in sufficient quantities to relieve pain, or withholding a painful course of (therapeutic) injections, even though by so doing the length of life may be shortened (in practice it rarely is). This is sometimes called 'passive euthanasia,' but this is not a very good term.

4. Intentional ending of a patient's life by a lethal injection, i.e., 'active' euthanasia' or 'suicide by proxy'.

Some ethicists argue that there is no difference between the last two because the effect is similar and, if you are a teleologist, this might be your view. In fact, the results may not be the same because by taking action 3, the *possibility* of recovery has not been ruled out and surprises do happen. The deontologists would argue that the motive and act are different. In 'passive' euthanasia, the intention is to relieve symptoms and the death is a bi-product (see double effect, Chapter 11). Whereas the intention in active euthanasia is killing or assisting suicide for the purpose of relieving suffering rather than saving another human life.

Are there, then, any absolutes for which there are no extenuating circumstances? Richard Higginson in his book *Dilemmas* suggests that rape and torture are two acts that are always wrong whatever the circumstances. This is a good point for discussion.

Precedence and priority

Although there may be few, if any, absolutes, many ethical decisions involve deciding which ethical principles should have priority. For example, the euthanasia debate centres on whether autonomy should have precedence over the value of a life. Does the patient's right to decide his or her own fate override the very high value that we should put on human life? In practical ethics, it is this decision of priority of two apparently conflicting ethical principles which is often the key point of the debate and the decision, and further examples will be given in later chapters.

References and Further Reading

Clark H (1964). *Philosophy of Albert Schweitzer*. Methuen, London.
Dunstan, GR (1974). *The Artifice of Ethics*. SCM Press, London.
Higginson R (1988). *Dilemmas*. Hodder and Stoughton, London.

11 Diverging paths: the variable results of ethical decisions

In our wanderings through the ethical jungle, we have often had to make decisions at places where the paths divide. It is sometimes possible to see where the paths eventually lead but sometimes it is not. The pathway may branch again just round the corner, one branch leading to good results and the other to bad. There are several terms in medical ethics that need to be discussed, which are concerned with the effects of our decisions as opposed to the principles and motives that lie behind them.

No doubt many would like to hold on to two differing views rather than make a decision between them — a policy known as *syncretism*. This is rather like a person trying to walk along with one foot on each of two diverging branches of a path — eventually she falls off between the two (Fig. 11.1). Unfortunately, decisions have

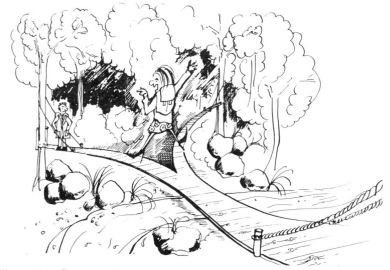

Figure 11.1 Syncretism!

to be made when paths diverge, but ethicists take comfort in two further doctrines.

The doctrine of double effect

This is particularly associated with Roman Catholic ethics. It states that an action, that is good, can be justified, even though it has a foreseen or unforeseen side-effect, which is bad. A classical example is the gynaecologist operating for an ectopic pregnancy to save a woman's life (which is good), but in order to do so he has to remove the pregnancy (which is bad). The good action is held to justify the bad. The same reasoning is used to justify so called 'passive euthanasia' where the 'good' act of relieving pain might lead to the 'bad' side-effect of shortening the patient's life. Such decisions are, indeed, very common in medical and surgical treatment, although usually the good and bad effects are probabilities rather than certainties. A double amputation of the legs to try to save a patient's life is a difficult decision, because there is no guarantee that his life will be saved, although it is known that he will die without the amputation. But if he does survive he will be condemned to a wheelchair existence. The doctrine, however, is usually used to refer to cases where life-saving action is involved.

The lesser of two evils

Unfortunately, in this imperfect world, the pressing decision is often not between the good act with a bad side-effect, but between two acts, neither of which is good. A choice has to be made between the lesser of two evils. The question of giving the contraceptive pill to a girl under 16 years who is having regular sexual relations with several partners is a common example.

To give the 'Pill' would be to agree to:
1.   Illegal sexual intercourse
2.   Risk of venereal disease and long-term risk of cervical cancer
3.   Risk of psychological/emotional problems later.

Not to give the 'Pill' would be to risk:
1.   An unwanted pregnancy
2.   Possible abortion with its physical and psychological sequelae
3.   An unwanted child to a very young mother.

The decision has to be made and weight given to the *seriousness* and *likelihood* of the various consequences. The weight given to each will depend on the particular doctor's moral code and experience.

The great problem with the 'lesser of two evils' policy is that after a time, familiarity leads to the lesser of two evils, no longer being regarded as evil, but as a good. The way to prevent that happening is to think through the reasons behind a particular action from time to time, and check that it can still be justified.

The corollary of the 'lesser of two evils' is the 'better of two goods'. Not all medical practice is concerned with the darker side of human nature. We wish to help a patient in two ways, the effects of which are mutually exclusive. Much of our practice involves this sort of decision, particularly when we are comparing physical and mental health.

The slippery slope

Sometimes the path we choose leads to a steep and slippery hill which we cannot see, and we find ourselves sliding down out of control (Fig. 11.2). How often have we heard the comment 'Don't do that, it is the thin edge of the wedge' or 'That piece of research is the top of a slippery slope'? Such comments refer to the feeling that once a course of action has been decided upon, it will inevitably lead to many unwanted effects, without anyone being able to control it. A clear stopping place cannot be foreseen and the consequences appear to be continuous.

New research in the field of *in vitro* fertilization is a good recent example. Once anyone was allowed to fertilize an ovum outside the mother, it was argued, there would be no stopping until we reached the full horror of a Brave New World with its cloning and control. This view sees science controlling of man, and man being unable to control science. The first is not true but the second may well be. The answer to dangerous knowledge is not necessarily more knowledge and man's use of other scientific discoveries such as atomic energy, is not very encouraging; but there is no reason, in principle, why statutory checks or voluntary checks should not be imposed. One of the concerns about *in vitro* fertilization research is that it should be limited to those couples who are married or in a long-term stable relationship so that the child will be properly cared for; this can easily be arranged if society and the gynaecologists wish. The second concern is about the fate of the many embryos that are not returned to the womb, because frequently more ova are fertilized than are needed. The Warnock Committee addressed this problem and decided that embryos should not be grown for more than two weeks (before the development of the primitive neural streak). Those who believe the unimplanted embryo is a full human being, did not accept this but they would be delighted by the news of recent techniques which are achieving as good pregnancy rates from a single fertilized ovum as from many. However, research workers of

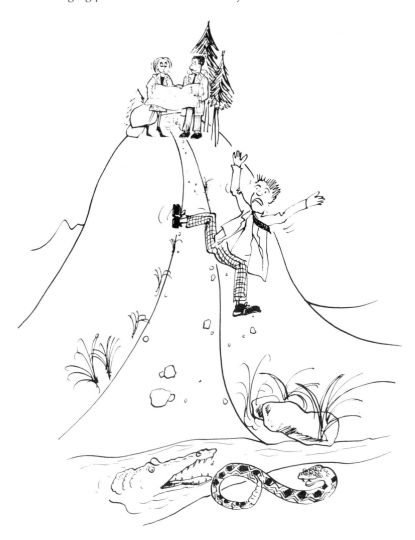

Figure 11.2 Is an ethical decision the start of a slippery slope?

all kinds must be prepared not to start research or even to abandon it, if its dangers appear to outweigh its benefits.

Even war has certain controls. Germ warfare has been outlawed in many countries and there is a convention for the treatment of prisoners of war. One of the anxieties over the legalization of euthanasia is that voluntary euthanasia could imperceptively slide into becoming semi-compulsory and then compulsory euthanasia (see Chapter 19).

Consistency

It is important to check that ethical decisions are consistent in different areas of medical practice. I am using the word 'consistent' in its general sense, not in its technical, philosophical, or mathematical sense. We have seen the inconsistency of telling relatives and not the patient about one disease but not another (p. 78). Another example is the acceptance, by some, of voluntary euthanasia for the dying patient to relieve the burden on his relatives; whereas the suggestion that a patient's kidney should be removed, even with relatives' permission, before he was dead, to improve the health of another patient, would be generally rejected as unethical. By the same token of consistency, experience gained from one area of practice can be a great help in guiding ethical decisions in a new area, as we will see in later examples.

All medical research has potential for abuse, or more correctly, all human beings have a potential to misuse scientific discoveries. That is why ethical discussion and committees are needed, and why students need to know about ethics.

References and Further Reading

Campbell AV and Higgs R (1982). *In that Case: Medical Ethics in Everyday Practice*. Darton Longman and Todd, London. (A vivid account of ethical decisions during the care of one patient and her family).
Warnock Committee (1984). *British Medical Journal;* **289**: 238–9.

12 The signposts on the way: ethical codes and ethical committees

Throughout this book we have often referred to various ethical codes. What role do they really have in shaping the practice of medicine? The problem is that no code can be at the same time rigid enough to live by, and elastic enough to meet all situations. Codes are sets of principles — rough guides — and have usually arisen when there has been a serious lapse in ethical standards, e.g., Thomas Percival's in the eighteenth century and the Declaration of Helsinki after the exposés at the Nuremberg trials, or when a completely new situation has arisen like the transplantation of cadaver organs (Declaration of Sydney). It is obviously impossible for doctors to think through the basis and implications of each decision, every day; they have to have what Professor Dunstan calls 'conventions' by which he means 'giving stability and permanence to a moral insight by embodying it in an institution, precisely because, without the institution, it is likely to be lost in time of need'; he points out that they do not rely primarily on the sanctions of the criminal law and that they are a community or group possession. In practice, they are adopted voluntarily by a profession or a country as the guidelines the group will aim to follow.

> Conventions are possible because men are capable of moral insight, of agreeing in the recognition of moral insight, and of committing themselves to maintain it; they rest on a presupposition of fidelity to a common interest and purpose. Conventions are necessary because men fail conspicuously to follow their moral insights and are capable of ruthlessly exploiting one another in the pursuit of self-interest; they rest on a presupposition of infidelity to the community purpose. And in this double statement, of possibility and necessity, stands the realism of ethics — and incidentally, the realism of Christian theology which sees man as both fallen and free, turned in upon self, while still ordained by nature and grace towards community and reconciliation with God
>
> *Artifice of Ethics*, p. 7

However, as we have seen in the previous chapters, conventions or codes are *second order* ethical statements that depend on the acceptance of the values that lie behind them. In Chapter 2 we saw that the Christians of the Middle Ages in Britain adopted the Hippocratic Oath from ancient Greece because most of it fitted with their own values and principles. We also saw how modern British society has neglected the clause on abortion, because the views of a large part of society have changed and no longer accept the values behind the convention or code. The weakness of codes when the underlying basis is not agreed, is shown by the very 'woolly' Declaration of Oslo. The only statements of any substances are:

1. Abortion should be performed only as a therapeutic measure [and that is vague enough]
2. A decision to terminate pregnancy should normally be approved in writing by at least two doctors chosen for their professional competence. [With that there must be agreement, but this says more about the way ethics are put into practice than about the ethics themselves.]

The Declaration of Helsinki is much more specific, because there is the general underlying agreement that the subject of the research should be protected by all possible safeguards, while allowing the research to continue for the benefit of others. The Declaration is concerned with methods rather than overall aims, which are agreed. However, conventions need not just be international codes. They can include the policy of a particular general practice or hospital department, that particular situations will be handled in an agreed way. The policy on telling patients their diagnosis is a good example of the way in which a convention can work. One department may have the convention that patients are not told — based on rejection of the principles of truth and patient autonomy, while another department may have an open policy. As conventions are a 'team' matter, it is important that they are discussed openly and agreed. So often the more junior members are seething inwardly about a policy dictated from the top. An association like the British Medical Association, through its central ethical committee, can develop practices that are adopted democratically and used as guidance. Many everyday decisions will be in categories that can be covered in this way. The ethical paths can often have clear signposts. The codes or conventions, however, are no substitute for the doctor's own conscience and he cannot merely hide behind the convention, especially when there is plenty of leeway and variation in practice (Fig. 12.1).

The well-known international codes are printed at the end of this chapter and not in the Appendix, because the appendices of most books are not read!

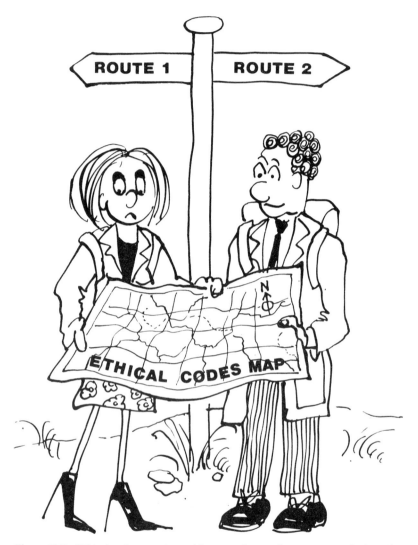

Figure 12.1 Ethical codes can give guidance on the way but are not a substitute for the individual conscience

Paul Ramsey (1970) comments as follows:

I do not believe that either the codes of medical ethics or the physicians who have undertaken to comment on them . . . will suffice to withstand the omnivorous appetite of scientific research or of a therapeutic technology that has a momentum and life of its own . . . 'codes' governing medical practice constitute a sort of 'catechism' in the ethics of the medical profession. These codes exhibit professional ethics which ministers and theologians and members of other professions can only profoundly respect and admire. Still a catechism never sufficed. Unless these principles are constantly pondered and enlivened in their application they become dead letters. There is also need that these principles be deepened and sensitised and opened to further humane revision in face of all the ordinary and the newly emerging situations which a doctor confronts — as do we all — in the present day.

Hospital Ethical Committees

These are now required in all hospitals and institutions where clinical research is performed (in the USA they are known as Institution Review Committees). They must have lay members as well as professional members, and all research protocols must be submitted to the ethical committee for approval before the research is started. Most grant-giving bodies require evidence that the proposed research has been approved by the local ethical committee before they will release the funding. Many submissions are routine, with no ethical problems, but sometimes the ethical committee can recommend changes in the design of a project, which can make it more ethical.

One of the great weaknesses of the system is that the committee is only obliged to see formal research projects. Any clinician is free to try a new treatment or perform a new operation on an individual patient without reference to the committee. The irony is that the doctor, who is prepared to admit that he is not sure which treatment is the best and submits two treatments to a formal trial has to obtain ethical committee approval and informed consent from the patient. The doctor who continues with an out-dated treatment, which he trusts, but which may be much worse than the modern treatment, can continue on his way without an ethical committee.

Trials of new drugs are approved by the Committee on Safety of Medicines (CSM) but the trial design will also be put before the local ethical committee. Ethical committees are not guarantors of complete safety but act as an added check to make sure that the enthusiastic research worker is not carried away, forgetting the ethical aspects of his plans. Yet at present in Britain, new procedures, artificial materials such as some sutures, and prostheses such as hip joints, do not have to be approved by a national committee before they are used on patients.

Research on children

Research on children presents particular problems of consent, because it has to be given by the parents on behalf of the child. The ethical committee has a very special part to play here and all applications for research involving children must be checked very carefully. It is not justified to use particularly invasive procedures, ionizing radiations and non-essential investigations which carry hazards.

Editorial Committees of Medical Journals

One important extra safeguard against unethical research is the medical journal in which the research worker hopes to publish his results. Most journals review papers from an ethical as well as a scientific standpoint and require acknowledgement on the paper that the research has passed a local ethical committee. But sometimes research turns out to be unethical, or becomes unethical once it has started and takes a turn that could not have been foreseen by the ethical committee at the start. The ethical research worker will stop and re-design his experiments or change direction altogether. The unethical research worker who continues, may only have the journal's editors as his final check. Late though this may be, if the work is turned down, the researcher will think again next time.

General ethical codes:

Hippocratic Oath

(*see* Chapter 2, p. 20)

Declaration of Geneva (Amended 1968)

At the time of being admitted as a Member of the Medical Profession:

I solemnly pledge myself to consecrate my life to the service of humanity;
I will give to my teachers the respect and gratitude which is their due;
I will practise my profession with conscience and dignity;
The health of my patient will be my first consideration;
I will respect the secrets which are confided in me, even after the patient has died;
I will maintain by all the means in my power, the honour and the noble traditions of the medical profession;
My colleagues will be my brothers;
I will not permit considerations of religion, nationality, race, party politics or social standing to intervene between my duty and my patients;
I will maintain the utmost respect for human life from the time of conception; even under threat, I will not use my medical knowledge contrary to the laws of humanity.
I make these promises solemnly, freely and upon my honour.

The International Code of Medical Ethics

Duties of Doctors in General

A DOCTOR MUST always maintain the highest standards of professional conduct.

A DOCTOR MUST practise his profession uninfluenced by motives of profit.

THE FOLLOWING PRACTICES are deemed unethical:

> (a) Any self advertisement except such as is expressly authorized by the national code of medical ethics.
> (b) Collaboration in any form of medical service in which the doctor does not have professional independence.
> (c) Receiving any money in connection with services rendered to a patient other than a proper professional fee, even with the knowledge of the patient.

ANY ACT OR ADVICE which could weaken physical or mental resistance of a human being may be used only in his interest.

A DOCTOR IS ADVISED to use great caution in divulging discoveries or new techniques of treatment.

A DOCTOR SHOULD certify or testify only to that which he has personally verified.

Duties of Doctors to the Sick

A DOCTOR MUST always bear in mind the obligation of preserving human life.

A DOCTOR OWES to his patient complete loyalty and all the resources of his science. Whenever an explanation or treatment is beyond his capacity he should summon another doctor who has the necessary ability.

A DOCTOR SHALL preserve absolute secrecy on all he knows about his patients because of the confidence entrusted in him.

A DOCTOR MUST give emergency care as a humanitarian duty unless he is assured that others are willing and able to give such care.

Duties of Doctors to Each Other

A DOCTOR OUGHT to behave to his colleagues as he would have them behave to him.

A DOCTOR MUST NOT entice patients from his colleagues.

A DOCTOR MUST OBSERVE the principles of The Declaration of Geneva approved by the World Medical Association.

Definitions of Death

The Declaration of Sydney (1968)

> (1) The determination of the time of death is in most countries the legal responsibility of the physician and should remain so. Usually he will be able without special assistance to decide that a person is dead, employing the classical criteria known to all physicians.
> (2) Two modern practices in medicine, however, have made it necessary to study the question of the time of death further: (i) the

ability to maintain by artificial means the circulation of oxygenated blood through tissues of the body which may have been irreversibly injured and (ii) the use of cadaver organs such as heart or kidneys for transplantation.

(3) A complication is that death is a gradual process at the cellular level with tissues varying in their ability to withstand deprivation of oxygen. But clinical interest lies not in the state of preservation of isolated cells but in the fate of a person. Here the point of death of the different cells and organs is not so important as the certainty that the process has become irreversible by whatever techniques of resuscitation that may be employed.

(4) This determination will be based on clinical judgment supplemented if necessary by a number of diagnostic aids of which the electroencephalograph is currently the most helpful. However, no single technological criterion is entirely satisfactory in the present state of medicine, nor can any one technological procedure be substituted for the overall judgment of the physician. If transplantation of an organ is involved, the decision that death exists should be made by two or more physicians and the physicians determining the moment of death should in no way be immediately concerned with the performance of the transplantation.

(5) Determination of the point of death of the person makes it ethically permissible to cease attempts at resuscitation and in countries where the law permits, to remove organs from the cadaver provided that prevailing legal requirements of consent have been fulfilled.

Memorandum issued by the Honorary Secretary of the Conference of Medical Royal Colleges and their Faculties in the United Kingdom (1979)

(1) In October 1976 the Conference of Royal Colleges and their Faculties (UK) published a report unanimously expressing the opinion that 'brain death', when it had occurred, could be diagnosed with certainty. The report has been widely accepted. The conference was not at that time asked whether or not it believed that death itself should be presumed to occur when brain death takes place, or whether it would come to some other conclusion. The present report examines this point and should be considered as an addendum to the original report.

(2) Exceptionally, as a result of massive trauma, death occurs instantaneously or near-instantaneously. Far more commonly, death is not an event: it is a process, the various organs and systems supporting the continuation of life failing and eventually ceasing altogether to function, successively and at different times.

(3) Cessation of respiration and cessation of the heart beat are examples of organic failure occurring during the process of dying, and since the moment that the heart beat ceases is usually detectable with simplicity by no more than clinical means, it has for many centuries been accepted as the moment of death itself, without any serious attempt being made to assess the validity of this assumption.

(4) It is now universally accepted, by the lay public as well as by the medical profession, that it is not possible to equate death itself with the cessation of the heart beat. Quite apart from the elective cardiac arrest of open-heart surgery, spontaneous cardiac arrest followed by successful resuscitation is today a common-place and although the more sensational accounts of occurrences of this kind still refer to the patient being 'dead' until restoration of the heart beat, the use of the quote marks usually demonstrates that this word is not to be taken literally, for to most people the one aspect of death that is beyond debate is its irreversibility.

(5) In the majority of cases in which a dying patient passes through the processes leading to the irreversible state we call death, successive organic failures eventually reach a point at which brain death occurs and this is the point of no return.

(6) In a minority of cases brain death does not occur as a result of the failure of other organs or systems but as a direct result of severe damage to the brain itself from, perhaps, a head injury or a spontaneous intracranial haemorrhage. Here the order of events is reversed: instead of the failure of such vital functions as heart beat and respiration eventually resulting in brain death, brain death results in the cessation of spontaneous respiration; and this is normally followed within minutes by cardiac arrest due to hypoxia. If, however, oxygenation is maintained by artificial ventilation, the heart beat can continue for some days, and haemoperfusion will for a time be adequate to maintain function in other organs, such as the liver and kidneys.

(7) Whatever the mode of its production, brain death represents the state at which a patient becomes truly dead, because by then all functions of the brain have permanently and irreversibly ceased. It is not difficult or illogical in any way to equate this with the concept in many religions of the departure of the spirit from the body.

(8) In the majority of cases, since brain death is part of or the culmination of a failure of all vital functions, there is no necessity for a doctor specifically to identify brain death individually before concluding that the patient is dead. In a minority of cases in which it is brain death that causes failure of other organs and systems, the fact that these systems can be artificially maintained even after death has made it important to establish a diagnostic routine which will identify with certainty the existence of brain death.

Conclusion
(9) It is the conclusion of the conference that the identification of brain death means that the patient is dead, whether or not the function of some organs, such as a heart beat, is still maintained by artificial means.

Clinical research and human experimentation

Declaration of Helsinki (Revised, 1975)

It is the mission of the medical doctor to safeguard the health of the people. His or her knowledge and conscience are dedicated to the fulfilment of this mission.

The Declaration of Geneva of the World Medical Association binds the doctor with the words, 'The health of my patient will be my first consideration', and the International Code of Medical Ethics declares that 'Any act or advice which could weaken physical or mental resistance of a human being may be used only in his interest.'

The purpose of biomedical research involving human subjects must be to improve diagnostic, therapeutic and prophylactic procedures and the understanding of the aetiology and pathogenesis of disease.

In current medical practice most diagnostic, therapeutic or prophylactic procedures involve hazards. This applies *a fortiori* to biomedical research.

Medical progress is based on research which ultimately must rest in part on experimentation involving human subjects.

In the field of biomedical research a fundamental distinction must be recognized between medical research in which the aim is essentially diagnostic or therapeutic for a patient, and medical research, the essential object of which is purely scientific and without direct diagnostic or therapeutic value to the person subjected to the research.

Special caution must be exercised in the conduct of research which may affect the environment, and the welfare of animals used for research must be respected.

Because it is essential that the results of laboratory experiments be applied to human beings to further scientific knowledge and to help suffering humanity, the World Medical Association has prepared the following recommendations as a guide to every doctor in biomedical research involving human subjects. They should be kept under review in the future. It must be stressed that the standards as drafted are only a guide to physicians all over the world. Doctors are not relieved from criminal, civil and ethical responsibilities under the laws of their own countries.

I *Basic Principles*

(1) Biomedical research involving human subjects must conform to generally accepted scientific principles and should be based on adequately performed laboratory and animal experimentation and on a thorough knowledge of the scientific literature.

(2) The design and performance of each experimental procedure involving human subjects should be clearly formulated in an experimental protocol which should be transmitted to a specially appointed independent committee for consideration, comment and guidance.

(3) Biomedical research involving human subjects should be conducted only by scientifically qualified persons and under the supervision of a clinically competent medical person. The responsibility for the human subject must always rest with the medically qualified person and never rest on the subject of the research, even though the subject has given his or her consent.

(4) Biomedical research involving human subjects cannot legitimately be carried out unless the importance of the objective is in proportion to the inherent risk to the subject.

(5) Every biomedical research project involving human subjects should be preceded by careful assessment of predictable risks in comparison with foreseeable benefits to the subject or to others. Concern for the interests of the subject must always prevail over the interests of science and society.

(6) The right of the research subject to safeguard his or her integrity must always be respected. Every precaution should be taken to respect the privacy of the subject and to minimize the impact of the study on the subject's physical and mental integrity and on the personality of the subject.

(7) Doctors should abstain from engaging in research projects involving human subjects unless they are satisfied that the hazards involved are believed to be predictable. Doctors should cease any investigation if the hazards are found to outweigh the potential benefits.

(8) In publication of the results of his or her research, the doctor is obliged to preserve the accuracy of the results. Reports of experimentation not in accordance with the principles laid down in this Declaration should not be accepted for publication.

(9) In any research on human beings, each potential subject must be adequately informed of the aims, methods, anticipated benefits and potential hazards of the study and the discomfort it may entail. He or she should be informed that he or she is at liberty to abstain from participation in the study and that he or she is free to withdraw his or her consent to participation at any time. The doctor should then obtain the subject's freely-given informed consent, preferably in writing.

(10) When obtaining informed consent for the research project, the doctor should be particularly cautious if the subject is in a dependent relationship to him or her or may consent under duress. In that case the informed consent should be obtained by a doctor who is not engaged in the investigation and who is completely independent of this official relationship.

(11) In case of legal incompetence, informed consent should be obtained from the legal guardian in accordance with national legislation. Where physical or mental incapacity makes it impossible to obtain informed consent, or when the subject is a minor, permission from the responsible relative replaces that of the subject in accordance with national legislation.

(12) The research protocol should always contain a statement of the ethical considerations involved and should indicate that the principles enunciated in the present Declaration are complied with.

II *Medical Research Combined with Professional Care*
(Clinical Research)
(1) In the treatment of the sick person, the doctor must be free to use a new diagnostic and therapeutic measure, if in his or her judgment it offers hope of saving life, re-establishing health or alleviating suffering.

(2) The potential benefits, hazards and discomfort of a new method

should be weighed against the advantages of the best current diagnostic and therapeutic methods.

(3) In any medical study, every patient — including those of a control group, if any — should be assured of the best proven diagnostic and therapeutic method.

(4) The refusal of the patient to participate in a study must never interfere with the doctor–patient relationship.

(5) If the doctor considers it essential not to obtain informed consent, the specific reasons for this proposal should be stated in the experimental protocol for transmission to the independent committee (I.2).

(6) The doctor can combine medical research with professional care, the objective being the acquisition of new medical knowledge, only to the extent that medical research is justified by its potential diagnostic or therapeutic value for the patient.

III *Non-Therapeutic Biomedical Research Involving Human Subjects (Non-clinical Biomedical Research)*

(1) In the purely scientific application of medical research carried out on a human being, it is the duty of the doctor to remain the protector of the life and health of that person on whom biomedical research is being carried out.

(2) The subjects should be volunteers — either healthy persons or patients for whom the experimental design is not related to the patient's illness.

(3) The investigator or the investigating team should discontinue the research if in his/her or their judgment it may, if continued, be harmful to the individual.

(4) In research on man, the interest of science and society should never take precedence over considerations related to the well-being of the subject.

Torture and other cruel, inhuman or degrading treatment or punishment in relation to detention and imprisonment.

Declaration of Tokyo (1975)

Preamble
It is the privilege of the medical doctor to practise medicine in the service of humanity, to preserve and restore bodily and mental health without distinction as to persons, to comfort and to ease the suffering of his or her patients. The utmost respect for human life is to be maintained even under threat, and no use made of any medical knowledge contrary to the laws of humanity.

Declaration
(1) The doctor shall not countenance, condone or participate in the practice of torture or other forms of cruel, inhuman or degrading procedures, whatever the offence of which the victim of such procedures is suspected, accused or guilty, and whatever the victim's beliefs or motives, and in all situations, including armed conflict and civil strife.

(2) For the purpose of this Declaration, torture is defined as the deliberate, systematic or wanton infliction of physical or mental suffering by one or more persons acting alone or on the orders of any authority, to force another person to yield information, to make a confession, or for any other reason.

(3) The doctor shall not provide any premises, instruments, substances or knowledge to facilitate the practice of torture or other forms of cruel, inhuman or degrading treatment or to diminish the ability of the victim to resist such treatment.

(4) The doctor shall not be present during any procedure during which torture or other forms of cruel, inhuman or degrading treatment is used or threatened.

(5) A doctor must have complete clinical independence in deciding upon the care of a person for whom he or she is medically responsible.

(6) Where a prisoner refuses nourishment and is considered by the doctor as capable of forming an unimpaired and rational judgment concerning the consequences of such a voluntary refusal of nourishment, he or she shall not be fed artificially. The decision as to the capacity of the prisoner to form such a judgment should be confirmed by at least one other independent doctor. The consequences of the refusal of nourishment shall be explained by the doctor to the prisoner.

(7) The World Medical Association will support, and should encourage the international community, the national medical associations and fellow doctors, to support the doctor and his or her family in the face of threats or reprisals resulting from a refusal to condone the use of torture or other forms of cruel, inhuman or degrading treatment.

(8) The doctor shall in all circumstances be bound to alleviate the distress of his fellow men, and no motive — whether personal, collective or political — shall prevail against this higher purpose.

Therapeutic abortion

Declaration of Oslo (1970)

(1) The first moral principle imposed upon the doctor is respect for human life as expressed in a clause of the Declaration of Geneva: 'I will maintain the utmost respect for human life from the time of conception'.

(2) Circumstances which bring the vital interests of a mother into conflict with the vital interests of her unborn child create a dilemma and raise the question whether or not the pregnancy should be deliberately terminated.

(3) Diversity of response to this situation results from the diversity of attitudes towards the life of the unborn child. This is a matter of individual conviction and conscience which must be respected.

(4) It is not the role of the medical profession to determine the attitudes and rules of any particular state or community in this matter, but it is our duty to attempt to ensure the protection of our patients and to safeguard the rights of the doctor within society.

(5) Therefore, where the law allows therapeutic abortion to be performed, or legislation to that effect is contemplated, and this is not against the policy of the national medical association, and where the legislature desires or will accept the guidance of the medical profession the following principles are approved:

(*a*) Abortion should be performed only as a therapeutic measure.

(*b*) A decision to terminate pregnancy should normally be approved in writing by at least two doctors chosen for their professional competence.

(*c*) The procedure should be performed by a doctor competent to do so in premises approved by the appropriate authority.

(6) If the doctor considers that his convictions do not allow him to advise or perform an abortion, he may withdraw while ensuring the continuity of (medical) care by a qualified colleague.

(7) This statement, while it is endorsed by the General Assembly of the World Medical Association, is not to be regarded as binding on any member association unless it is adopted by that member association.

References and Further Reading

Dunstan GR (1974). *The Artifice of Ethics*. SCM Press, London.

Ramsay P (1976). *The Patient as Person*. Yale University Press, New Haven, Connecticut and London.

Royal College of Physicians (1990). *Guidelines on the practice of ethics committees in medical research involving human subjects* (2nd edition). Royal College of Physicians of London.

Royal College of Physicians (1990). *Research involving patients*. Royal College of Physicians of London.

Short D (1987). The future of local ethical research committees. *Journal of the Royal College of Physicians*. London, **21**: 67–9.

In September 1989, the World Medical Association met in Hong Kong and issued a number of Declarations and Statements some of which are referenced under the relevant chapters: Declaration of Hong Kong on abuse of the elderly. Statement on the persistent vegetative state.

13 Perimeter fences: the place of law

Law and ethics are closely related and in some medical schools ethics is discussed in the context of the course in forensic medicine. The proper functioning of the law, like ethical medical practice, depends on the acceptance by the community of the moral basis for the laws. If a majority of people believes that stealing is right and good, it will be very difficult to enforce a law against it, especially with a jury. Enforcement of law without consensus of agreement becomes tyranny. What then can the law do to enforce, uphold, or encourage ethical medical practice? First of all we must look at its limitations.

Limitation of law

The limitations of law are as follows:

1. It can only set limits to guarantee a minimum standard. That is why the designation 'perimeter fence' has been used for this chapter. The law is a fence to stop people straying too far from the right path (Fig. 13.1), but it cannot *guarantee* good behaviour. It cannot be a positive incentive to improve ethical performance and is a blunt instrument to solve ethical problems. To legislate for every individual action may not only be unworkable but also unfair to minority groups.

2. The law cannot make a judgment of a hypothetical case in advance. The doctor cannot expect a judge to give a definite answer to the question 'What would be the opinion of the law if I took such and such an action?' Because so much British practice is based on *case law* the reply would be 'I can only tell you when a similar case has been to court and I have seen what the court decides.' A good example of this testing of the law is discussed below (Dr Arthur case). Unfortunately, proceedings did not clarify the grey areas of the law as it had been hoped, but

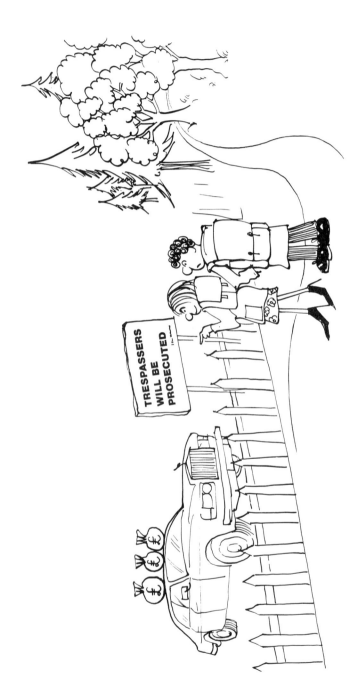

Figure 13.1   The Law acts as a perimeter fence to limit unethical behaviour

someone had to bring a case to court with all its expense and trauma for the law to give a judgment.

3. The working of law usually allows varying interpretations. Drafting of law is a highly skilled business. Laws must not be so cumbersome that they are impracticable or so vague that they are unenforceable. The 1967 Abortion Act illustrates this well. Whatever the original intention of the Act, it has led to abortion on request in many parts of the country. It is so loosely worded that it can be interpreted very freely. One clause states that the abortion can be performed '. . . if continuation of the pregnancy causes a risk greater than if the pregnancy were terminated'. (This was not in the original draft but was added later.) With modern safe methods of abortion, it can nearly *always* be said the continuation of the pregnancy carries more risk to the mother than the abortion at an early stage, even if the difference may be a risk of 0.1 per cent, compared with 0.2 per cent. This loose wording, whether intentional or not, has opened the way effectively to liberal abortion.

In the area of euthanasia, Lord Raglan, after the defeat of his Euthanasia Bill in the House of Lords, wrote in 1972:

> I have come to the conclusion after three years and hearing criticisms of it, that it may well be an insuperable problem to draw up a suitable declaration.

A special panel appointed by the Board of Science and Education of the British Medical Association (1971) concluded:

> . . . after careful consideration the Panel is convinced that it would be impossible to provide adequate safeguards in any euthansia legislation.

Since this statement, at least one country — Holland — has tried to introduce legislation and it remains to be seen, if it is passed, whether safeguards are effective. But whatever one's views on the rightness or wrongness of legislation, the law has a real problem in ensuring the intended aims are carried out and safeguarded.

The role of law

What then can the law achieve? The law can:

1. *Set clearly defined limits* For example, the law can legislate for unlawful killing and murder and it can legislate for a definition of death. It can deal with gross examples of professional misconduct through bodies such as the General Medical Council (GMC). It can define consent under well-defined

conditions, such as a surgical operation or clinical research, and it can legislate about confidentiality, such as access to medical records. Laws have been made, as we have seen, to attempt to regulate abortion and forbid surrogacy.

2. *Decide on who makes decisions*   The law can establish statutory bodies such as the GMC to oversee professional ethics and it can ensure that the framework exists to approve research projects by ethical committees, but the actual working and decisions of these bodies is left to the individual organizations. The law can also lay down rules about the giving and taking of medical evidence. The setting up of Community Health Councils provides a forum for patients to give advice and express concern about medical practice.

3. *Restrict a patient's autonomy*   We have already seen in Chapter 8, that the law has the power to restrict an individual's freedom under certain conditions. The isolation of patients with infectious diseases and the compulsory detention of patients in mental institutions are the main examples. John Stuart Mill, with his utilitarian philosophy, believed that the law should only restrict the freedom of the individual for the sake of others. However, it is difficult to foresee whether the effect of an action will remain limited in this way. When the Wolfenden Committee in the 1950s recommended that homosexual acts between consenting adults in private should no longer be a criminal offence, it did not foresee the AIDS epidemic of the 1980s. It is also worth noting that consent in this context does not carry the same safeguards of autonomy as consent to medical treatment (Chapter 8), and there is no guarantee that people are not being infected against their will and therefore losing their autonomy.

    The law also gives the right to restrict freedom for someone's own good, e.g., compulsory detention in mental institutions and compulsory wearing of seat-belts. Although law is a bad instrument for protecting people against themselves, it may have to be used in certain situations.

4. It can establish lines of responsibility and accountability. This is done by laws of contract, the role of defence organizations and family practitioner committees. The law can also provide a framework for patients to obtain redress by litigation and through a complaints procedure, both local and national, by the Health Service Commissioner (Ombudsman).

    This introduces the other area where the law has an increasing influence in the way medicine is practiced, namely litigation. Is litigation a good way of controlling unethical practice?

Litigation

Litigation against doctors has reached terrifying proportions in the USA and now probably works to the detriment of the patients rather than to their benefit. The reasons that the problem is so great in the USA are threefold:

1. The large number of lawyers who need an income. It is estimated that one-third of the lawyers who have ever practised in the history of the world are practising in the USA today!
2. The system of payment whereby the lawyer can take a proportion of the damages and so the higher the damage, the more he benefits; and the patient need pay no legal fees.
3. The high fees that many doctors have charged encourages the attitude in patients that unless the result is perfect, they will demand some of their money back.

Within the context of British medicine, litigation is unlikely to reach such proportions, but in 1987 we saw our first million pound settlement for damages for a private neurosurgical operation that went wrong. Lawyers in Britain are not allowed to take a proportion of the damages as their fees and as most patients are not paying directly for their treatment, they do not have the same financial incentive to sue. But lawyers in Britain are turning increasingly to medical litigation as a means of livelihood and the general public are becoming more aware of their rights in law. Litigation is increasing both in its frequency and in the size of settlements, as is indicated by the recent exponential rise in subscription to the Medical Defence Societies (but they are still only a fraction of the premiums in the USA). Let us look briefly at the role of litigation on the British scene, and it is worth noting, in passing, that lawyers divide medical practice into three broad categories: diagnosis, advice and treatment. (*See* comment on p. 114).

The benefits and dangers of litigation

Some might argue that the best way to deal with unethical behaviour would be to let the patient settle it through the courts. They would say that only the worst cases of malpractice come to the established ethical bodies, such as the GMC. The problem is that most of the cases of litigation are not concerned with ethical problems but with technical problems. Many of the cases that patients wish to bring are about personal, sometimes trivial matters and the important issues are untouched. Once a person acquires a litigious mentality he may lose all sense of proportion. It is reported that, in the USA, a man failed to pass the entrance examination to university, so sued his obstetrician for possible brain damage at birth 19 years before, although his high school record had been perfectly sound! A third disadvantage is that whether or not a case is brought to court depends on the chances of winning that case. Despite legal aid, to some extent, this still depends on the patient's ability to pay his costs if he loses. One good effect that litigation has had in the USA is that doctors have had to be far more honest with their patients about their diagnoses and the *expectations* and risks of treatments.

A patient must have the right to sue his doctor under civil law; but, in practice, frequent litigation leads to defensive and wasteful medicine, such as reluctance to introduce even well-tried new treatments, and many unnecessary expensive investigations. It also strains the relationship between doctor and patient and the doctor cannot ever say to his patient he is sorry that something has gone wrong, in case that implies his responsibility for it. In addition, there are two other weaknesses; firstly, a patient who shouts loudly, but does not necessarily have the best case, reaches court, whereas those with a justifiable claim often do not know how to obtain compensation. Secondly, compensation depends on proving negligence by a person or persons. This is the greatest weakness for the patients, as they do not receive compensation for what was a pure accident. It is for these reasons that at least two countries — New Zealand and Sweden — have introduced 'No fault compensation', where a patient does not have to prove negligence but presents his case to a tribunal where a decision and settlement of the scale of damages is made out of court. The patient still has the right to sue if she wishes, and matters of ethical, as opposed to technical failure can still be reported to the appropriate disciplinary bodies. Unfortunately, in New Zealand, the indications for allowable compensations have been made too wide, which is leading to the system falling into disrepute and becoming very expensive.

Important legal cases — ruling and guidelines

Throughout the last fifty years, there have been legal cases which have had extensive publicity and have sometimes clarified ethical guidelines and sometimes not. There has also been some specific legislation concerned with medical ethical matters. It must be remembered that whenever a specific case has been discussed, the details of the law are different in different countries and a judgment in one cannot automatically be transferred to the other.

Cases relating to death and prolonging life

Dr Bodkin Adams

In 1957, Dr Adams, a general practitioner from the south coast of England, was charged with murder. The trial took place seven years after an elderly widow with a stroke had died while under his care. She had been addicted to opiates for the previous two years, and Dr Adams increased the doses of the drug and added another sedative over the last week of her life. It came to light that the patient had altered her will in his favour and by her death he stood to make considerable financial gain (Fig. 13.1). After a prolonged trial in which some other medical reputations were tarnished, due to overdramatization in the witness box, the jury declared him not guilty of murder but guilty of failure to keep an accurate record of his use of dangerous drugs. They concluded, therefore, that he was unwise and careless rather than criminal. They were unconvinced that he intended to kill her, although he had a good motive, and were unconvinced that giving the larger doses of opiates (no larger than are given to many patients who are terminally ill) was the direct cause of her death. He was unwise in not handing the care of the patient over to a colleague once he realized that he was a beneficiary under her will. The very fact that he was charged with murder upheld the law on active involuntary euthanasia but the fact that he was acquitted was a great relief to many doctors whose patients died while under their care and whose pain had been controlled with large doses of morphine or heroin (*see* passive euthanasia, p. 83; and the principle of double effect, p. 86).

Karen Quinlan

A 21-year-old girl was admitted unconscious to hospital in the USA in April 1975 and for months she lay paralysed (but with a small area of residual brain activity) supported by an artificial respirator and with a gastric feeding tube. In October her parents applied to the courts for permission for the respirator to be switched off, but the physicians and State Attorney General refused. This raised three questions, as Ian Kennedy pointed out at the time: first, the definition of death; second, autonomy and the 'right to die' and third, the aims of treatment and the extent of a doctor's obligation to his patient. It also brought into sharp focus the role of the law courts, and whether guidelines drawn up by the profession and public, or case law, is the best way of establishing the right code of practice.

The New Jersey Supreme Court, which overruled the State Attorney's judgment, decided that every individual had the right to refuse medical care and this right still existed for incompetent patients. Her father was granted full power to make decisions for her. The Court also established an analytical framework for this and similar decisions in the future, which asked five questions:

1. Is there a right to terminate care?
2. What type of care can be terminated?
3. From what types of patients can care be terminated?
4. Who should act as decision-maker?

5. What are appropriate criteria for justifying the termination of medical care?

EJ Emanuel (1988) (qv) has written an excellent review based on this case.

Dr Leonard Arthur

In 1981, members of the pro-life organization 'Life' instigated legal proceedings against a paediatrician, Dr Arthur, who had looked after a newborn baby suffering from Down's Syndrome and rejected by her mother. As in the case of Dr Adams, he was charged with murder because he prescribed quite large doses of dihydrocodeine for sedative purposes.

Otherwise the baby received nursing care only and no special efforts were made to keep her alive when she developed serious complications. Unlike Dr Adams, Dr Arthur would receive no financial benefit from his patient's death and all were agreed that he was a caring, compassionate doctor. After a rather unsatisfactory trial with eminent witnesses appearing on behalf of the defendant and some rather dubious production of last minute pathological evidence, which had not been shown to the Crown pathologist, Dr Arthur was acquitted because there was sufficient doubt whether the drug had actually caused the baby's death. As a result of this confusion, the case did not resolve the issue of passive euthanasia, as those who had initiated the proceedings had hoped.

But it is worth asking whether Dr Arthur was given special consideration by the court because he was a doctor and whether, if the *parents* had taken the baby home and treated her in this way, even for the best of motives, they would have been acquitted?

Cases relating to negligence, consent and confidentiality

The Bolam Test

In 1957, Mr Justice McNair was presiding in the case of a claim for damage by a patient named Bolam who had undergone ECT treatment in Friern Barnet Hospital. The Court ruled that the doctor could not be found negligent if he could show that he was following current medical practice. This principle has guided similar cases since then but it is beginning to be questioned.

The Willowbrook Affair

Willowbrook was a large residential hospital for the care of subnormal people. A research project was instigated aimed at improving the infective hepatitis which was endemic in the hospital. The method to be used was to administer the virus to subnormal children. The justification being that they might get the infection anyway and it would be better for them to contract the infection under controlled conditions, which could then be studied.

This case caused a tremendous outcry. The key point in the discussion was not only concerned with whether patients should be given a virus intentionally, but also whether informed consent had been obtained from the parents. Many of them claimed that they had not had the research explained to them carefully and they had not given free individual consent because they were subject to pressure.

The Sidaway Case

Mrs Sidaway was an elderly woman who had an operation for a slipped disc but was left with damage to the spinal cord, causing some paralysis of her arm. She claimed damages of £67 500 for negligence by the neurosurgeon on the grounds of failure to disclose or to explain to her the risks of the operation. The surgeon had died, so there was no direct evidence about what he had actually told her. Mr Justice Skinner rejected the claim and five Law Lords dismissed an appeal, but Lord Scarman gave a dissenting judgment, which he discussed in a paper to the Royal Society of Medicine (1986).

Although this case clearly rejected the type of detailed consent for operation that is normal in the USA (Brahams D, 1984), it has acted as a warning to doctors to consider and document carefully, the explanations that are given to patients before they give consent, and it has strengthened the case for a more detailed surgical consent form.

The Gillick Case

Mrs Victoria Gillick challenged in court the guidelines issued in 1980 to doctors by the Department of Health and Social Security (DHSS) which stated '. . . A doctor was entitled in exceptional circumstances to prescribe contraceptives to a girl under 16 years-old in England and Wales without the consent of the parents'. The grounds of her case were that the doctors would be accessories to the crime of unlawful sexual intercourse and that the policy infringed the rights of parents over their children. The court upheld the DHSS guidelines but the Court of Appeal reversed the decision and confirmed the existing law that the parents were responsible for decisions affecting their children and the child herself did not have autonomy in this matter. In 1985, the Law Lords reversed the decision again and supported the DHSS against Mrs Gillick.

Professor Kennedy, commenting on the original case, pointed out that the doctor would only be an accessory to the crime of unlawful sexual intercourse if he prescribed the contraceptive pill *in collusion* with the male partner. The Law Lords gave five special circumstances in which doctors were justified in prescribing the Pill to a minor without telling her parents. These are that the girl:
1. Understands the implications
2. Cannot be persuaded to tell her parents
3. Is likely to begin or continue sexual intercourse without contraceptives
4. Unless she receives treatment, will suffer damage to her health
5. Her best interests are served by treatment without parental knowledge.

When these exceptions are studied, it will be seen that clauses (1), (2) and (3) will nearly always apply. Clause (4) is always true, as pregnancy in a 15-year-old will affect her health adversely. (5) is a difficult clause and depends on the doctors knowing the likely reaction of the patient's parents and making a fine judgment. Suggested guidelines issued during this prolonged trial, and appeal, were confused and even suggested that the doctor would be liable for prosecution if he did tell the parents and, indeed, applied the existing law. The latest guidelines of the DHSS in 1986 state:

> '*exceptionally* in cases where persuasion to tell the parent fails, the doctor should be free to prescribe without parental knowledge.

This is an interesting case in several respects. First, there is the important observation that judges could not agree and the verdicts were altered twice at different stages of the appeal. Secondly, it is an example of the employer, the DHSS, giving ethical guidelines to doctors. Thirdly, however, the case gave the Law Lords the opportunity and responsibility to state the exceptions to a general ethical rule. Their ruling has not given doctors *carte blanche* to prescribe the Pill to under-age girls under all circumstances. Fourthly, nevertheless, we can see on careful analysis that the exceptions can be fulfilled in nearly every case. The law makes the framework, but the assessment and final decision is left with the doctor.

Reports and recommendations relating to embryo research and conception

The Warnock Committee
The Warnock Committee was established in July 1982 with the following terms of reference:

> . . .to consider recent and potential developments in medicine and science relating to human fertilization and embryology; to consider what policies and safeguards should be applied including consideration of the social, ethical and legal implications of these developments and to make recommendations.

It reported two years later (*BMJ* (1984); **289**: 238) and made a number of recommendations on the making of laws and setting up of a new statutory licensing authority to control research and infertility services. Interestingly, there was not unanimous agreement on either the use of spare embryos for research or whether embryos should be created specially for research. The Committee recommended legal protection for the embryo in broad terms and also a number of alterations to the existing laws. It also discussed the legal aspects of inheritance for children conceived in various ways.

The Warnock Committee illustrates the use of law in ethics. Law can produce some broad rules and can set up the framework for monitoring — in this case, a licensing authority. But as we have seen elsewhere, it has to leave the individual decision to that authority. It also illustrates that on the most contentious issues there is strong disagreement and the proportion holding each view will depend largely on the way the committee is selected.

Surrogacy

Surrogacy, where one woman bears a child for another is an important question. The embryo is either fertilized *in vitro* from the sperm and egg of another couple and then implanted in the surrogate mother's uterus or the surrogate mother is fertilized with the sperm of the husband of the couple with the underlying promise that the child will be returned to them. The surrogate mother's uterus is being used as an 'incubator' on behalf of another woman. Regulation was urgent at the time of the Warnock Committee because profit-making agencies were just starting in Britain. Warnock recommended legislation to make it a criminal offence to set up or operate surrogate agencies, commercial or otherwise. Individuals entering into private surrogate arrangements would not be liable to criminal prosecution. This legislation was passed as the Surrogacy Arrangements Act in 1985 and it shows that the law is good at dealing with public and private agencies but can do little about local private arrangements. The whole debate raises two important ethical principles: one is the well-discussed matter of the value of the embryo and at what point it becomes fully human; the other is the question of autonomy and right. There is often an implicit assumption that it is the right of all couples to have children, even though, for example, the woman's Fallopian tubes may have been blocked by previous sexually transmitted infection. Where does this right come from? Is infertility any different from other bodily malfunctions which medicine tries to relieve with methods which are ethically controlled?

The Warnock Committee took extensive evidence over two years from many different groups and organizations and the same organizations were asked to make comments on its findings. This well-conducted and thoroughly researched study illustrates both the problems of legislation and of the recommending of ethical guidelines in a pluralistic society. Even those who disagree with

---

In April 1990, the House of Commons passed two bills: (i) to legalise the Warnock Committee recommendation that research on human embryos should be allowed up to 14 days' gestation; (ii) to reduce the upper limit for legal abortion from 28 weeks' to 24 weeks' gestation.

some of the findings cannot fault the thoroughness and sensitivity of the deliberations.

References and Further Reading

Brahams D (1984). The surgeon's duty to warn of risks. Transatlantic approach rejected by Court of Appeal. *Lancet;* **1**: 578–9.
Emanuel EJ (1988). A review of ethical and legal aspects of terminating medical care. *American Journal of Medicine;* **84**: 291–301.
Hawkins C (1985). *Mishap or Malpractice?*. Blackwells Scientific Publications, Oxford and London.
Kennedy IM (1976). The Karen Quinlan case: problems and proposals. *Journal of Medical Ethics;* **2**: 3–7.
Professional Standards (1972). BMA, London.
Raglan, Lord (1972). The problem of euthanasia. *Contact* Suppl. **38**.
Scarman, Lord (1986). Consent, communication and responsibility. *Journal of the Royal Society of Medicine;* **76**: 697–700.

Very recently in Britain, hospitals have agreed to carry the insurance against litigation for doctors treating NHS patients.

Part 2
Pathways in practice

Introduction

In the second part of this book, the methods of analysis, principles and algorithms which have been discussed in the previous chapters, are now applied to individual situations. These have been chosen in order to illustrate a wide variety of subjects and to focus on topics which will be particularly important over the next few years. I have purposely not tried to cover all the common ethical problems, although many have been used to illustrate the earlier chapters. Six topics are used to show how the ethical issues can be worked out. The aim of this book has been to encourage readers to find out the answers for themselves, rather than to provide ready-made solutions, because details of the problems rapidly change. Once students are familiar with common ethical components and arguments, they will not need to travel down formal pathways everytime they make a decision. Exactly the same transition occurs in clinical diagnosis when, after a time, a student can come to the right conclusion without going through the detailed descriptions that he learnt in the introductory course. Many everyday decisions will appear to be commonsense. But like many 'commonsense' legal judgments, they must be checked regularly against basic principles and the decisions justified.

The final chapter points out the importance of making choices, because that is what ethics — and life in general — must involve. My hope is that by the time that readers have reached the end of the book, they will have worked out the principles and bases of their own ethics and will be equipped to make the choices that will face them everyday in clinical practice. The full algorithm is repeated at the opening of chapter 14.

14 Should I tell my patient she has cancer?

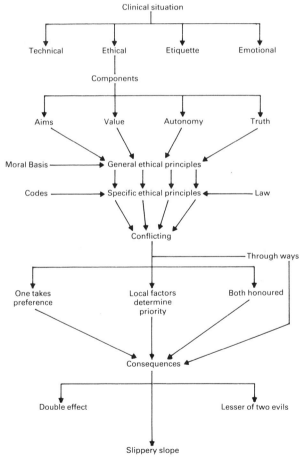

Clinical situation

Technical   Ethical   Etiquette   Emotional

Components

Aims   Value   Autonomy   Truth

Moral Basis ⟶ General ethical principles

Codes ⟶ Specific ethical principles ⟵ Law

Conflicting

Through ways

One takes preference   Local factors determine priority   Both honoured

Consequences

Double effect   Lesser of two evils

Slippery slope

Figure 14.1

This is a common, but difficult, ethical problem facing doctors in caring for patients, and it also has important implications for nursing staff and other health workers directly involved in patient care. We will use the pathway diagram on the previous page to analyse and try to resolve this problem.

Is there an ethical issue?

There is undoubtedly an ethical issue because the decision is concerned with truth, and with the life and death of the patient. But there is also a considerable emotional element, not only for the patient but also for the doctor. Sometimes doctors decide not to tell a patient in order to avoid being embarrassed by the tearful reaction. No one with any sensitivity finds it easy to tell a patient she is going to die; but it is wrong if the desire to protect himself from emotional distress becomes more important to the doctor than telling the truth for the ultimate good of his patient (Fig. 14.2).

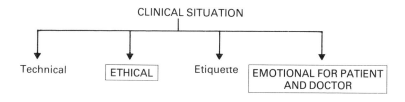

Figure 14.2

The ethical components

In this case, the ethical decision involves three areas: (*see* fig. 14.3).

1. The aims of medical care and benefit for the patient
2. The patient's, doctor's and relative's autonomy
3. Truth and integrity.

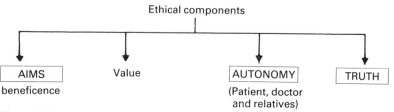

Figure 14.3

What are the ethical principles and their basis?

Aims of medical care

The general ethical principles that govern this decision are the duties to benefit the patient and to do no harm. It is important to decide what is meant by 'good' and by 'harm'. The immediate reaction of the patient will probably be one of anger and distress, but in the long term it may be better for her to be able to adjust to her progressive weakness, arrange her financial affairs and sort out any problems with the family. Deception overcomes the short-term distress at the expense of accumulating long-term problems for both the patient and the family. The aim of telling her the truth is still to help her in the long term (Fig 14.4).

Autonomy

The patient has the right to know or not to know about the disease. A few doctors might suggest that it is *their* right to tell the patient what they like, but, as discussed in Chapter 9, it is the *patient's illness and she should be the arbiter of what she wants to know*. On the other hand, the family has some autonomy too, and what the patient is told also affects them. The doctor's autonomy gives him the right not to be forced by relatives to tell the patient a lie. Relatives not infrequently try to persuade doctors into this decision.

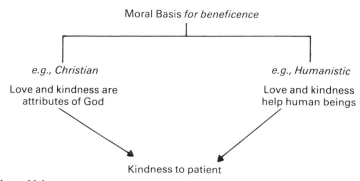

Figure 14.4

Truth and integrity

Telling the truth, as we have seen in Chapter 9, is one of the most important ethical principles for those with a strong theistic moral basis (Fig. 14.5). For some it is overriding, with no exceptions, but for others, although it is still very important, it can be broken under certain extenuating circumstances. On the other hand, for a few people with a teleological outlook on ethics, truth is not important in itself but only matters if it produces the right consequences for the patient and her family. So, these doctors or nurses may still tell the truth as a means to an end but will be happy to refrain from telling it, or to tell a lie, if that appears to achieve more immediate happiness.

Specific Ethical Principles

So to summarize, the specific ethical principles in this case are that the:

1. Aim is to benefit the patient and her family in the long-term, to be as kind to her as possible and give her minimal distress.
2. Patient's autonomy and her right to know the truth must be respected.
3. Family's autonomy and involvement in the illness must be respected.
4. Doctor's autonomy gives him the right not to be asked to tell a lie by pressure from the relatives or from the patient.
5. Truth must be told and integrity maintained in relation to the patient.

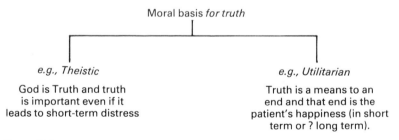

Figure 14.5

Ethical codes and law

Do the ethical codes or law help in this decision? The ethical codes say very little about telling the truth to the patient. The law would come in if the doctor had deceived the patient, who had then made some business transaction or financial arrangements assuming he was going to live for a long time. In the USA, the fear of litigation is a strong spur to truth-telling.

Do these principles conflict?

What conflicts can occur between any of these principles? One way to resolve them is for the truth to be a 'through-way' — 'the truth, the whole truth and nothing but the truth', anything else being subordinated to this overriding principle (Fig. 14.6). It is neither ethically nor legally right that relatives should be able to prevent a patient of sound mind being told the truth and the relative's autonomy must be subordinated to that of the patient and the doctor. However, there may be special circumstances — for example, in an elderly patient who is very confused — where relatives should be told first and the patient herself not told at that time (Fig. 14.7). The conflict of the patient's autonomy and truth is resolved by the patient being given the opportunity and encouragement to ask as much as she wants to know, rather than having the truth thrust on her. The conflict of truth and benefit is overcome by the *way* the patient is told — gradually and with compassion, so that she can adjust to the news and be supported and helped to come to terms with it.

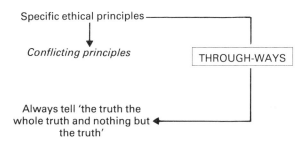

Figure 14.6

Consequences

There may be seen and unseen consequences to these decisions. Very occasionally, a patient reacts most adversely to the news and takes her own life or 'turns her face to the wall and gives up the will to live'. The action in telling could still be considered justified under the principle of double effect, in that this was a possible risk, but not a direct result of the action. If suicide was considered to be very likely, from knowledge of the patient's mental state, then this might justify withholding some part of the truth but not in telling a direct lie (*see* discussion on p. 73). The figures show, in diagrammatic form, how the decisions were made and resolved (Figs. 14.6–14.8)

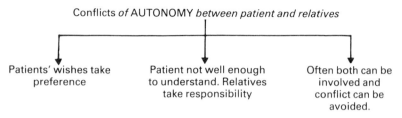

Figure 14.7

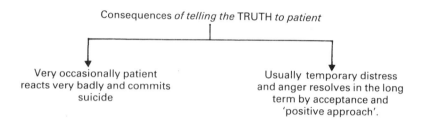

Figure 14.8

What happens in practice

Figure 14.9 shows the results of the survey performed in Sheffield about what actually happens and who is told what. This was taken by Wilkes in 1983 and, even since then, attitudes have changed probably more in favour of giving the patients more and more information about their illness.

	General practitioner	Hospital doctors	Hospital nurses
Whole truth (%)	27	20	5
Part of truth (%)	26	28	7
Lies (%)	5	3	1
Nothing (%)	33	24	61
Patient unfit (%)	8	25	25

Figure 14.9   Who tells what?

(Reproduced with permission from Wilkes, E. (Ed.) (1986). *A Source Book of Terminal Care.* Sheffield University Printing Unit, Sheffield)

References and Further Reading

Kubler-Ross E (1969). *On Death and Dying*. McMillan, New York.

Saunders Cicely MS (1977). Telling patients. In Reiser SJ, Dyck AJ and Curran WJ, *Ethics in Medicine*. MIT Press, London.

Twycross R (1985). *The Dying Patient*. Christian Medical Fellowship, London.

15 The ethical problems of AIDS

The Acquired Immune Deficiency Syndrome (AIDS) — the florid manifestation of infection with the human immuno deficiency virus (HIV) — is a new problem in Britain and has raised a host of urgent ethical questions. There has not been time to draw up an international declaration on AIDS (even if that were appropriate), and we have had to think through the issues directly. It is, therefore, a very good example to test the thesis of this book: that an established algorithm can be used to face new situations.

Are there ethical questions and if so, what are they?

Because AIDS is incurable and infectious and related to sexual behaviour, it is very emotive. It is important to try to identify emotional bias when analysing these problems. There are also large political overtones in their widest sense: government involvement, international relationships with African countries, and gay rights movements all tend to confuse the picture. The one technical concern is the accuracy of the screening test. There are at least three ethical problems. Should:

1. Patients, their sexual partners and their relatives be told of the diagnosis?
2. Asymptomatic people be screened?
3. The freedom of AIDS sufferers be restricted in some way to protect other people?

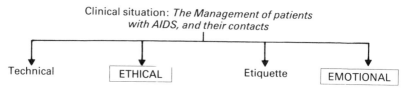

Figure 15.1

What are the ethical components?

Telling the patients, partners and relatives is in the realm of *truth-telling* and *confidentiality*. Screening and isolation are concerned with *autonomy* and *confidentiality*. There is little conflict over the *aims* of treatment, which are to care for the patient in every possible way and to prevent the spread of the disease to others.

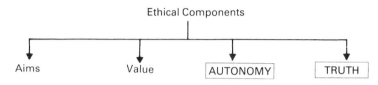

Figure 15.2

The ethical principles in telling the patient the diagnosis

Informing a patient that he is suffering from AIDS is very similar to informing a patient that he has inoperable cancer, although the life expectancy may be far longer with AIDS. Because of all the publicity, euphemisms cannot be used, even if they were desirable. The decision rests between telling him and providing the necessary counselling and support, or telling a lie with all its consequences (see below), or just remaining silent.

There is increasing evidence that it is in the patient's interest for him and his doctor to know he has the disease. For example, the potentially overwhelming chest infections can be treated with antibiotics as soon as they start. A mother who knows she has HIV infection may be able to prevent her newborn baby being infected from her milk, if she does not breast-feed. On the other hand, the patient's autonomy gives him the right not to know if his ignorance does not harm others, even if it is detrimental to himself. But in many moral systems it is good and right to protect other lives, even at inconvenience to oneself.

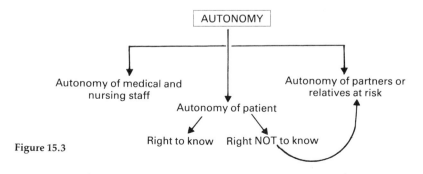

Figure 15.3

Confidentiality and autonomy

There is a fundamental difference, however, between AIDS and cancer, in that AIDS is infectious, in certain ways, whereas most cancers are not. Furthermore, a present or future partner is at risk. Therefore, whereas doctors might not necessarily tell the patient's spouse that he has cancer, it might be very important to tell her that he has AIDS or is HIV-positive, for her protection and the protection of their children, present or future. Unfortunately, she may already be infected before she learns that he has the virus. The question is this: 'Is this an exception to the principle of confidentiality, because the consequences are so serious?' The doctor's duty is very strong to persuade the patient to tell his partner, but his chances of succeeding depend on the closeness of the doctor/patient relationship. The doctor may also need to notify the health authorities, although AIDS is not yet a notifiable disease in Britain in the same way as typhoid or polio. The final question is whether the doctor has the right to impose his sexual ethic on the patient or whether this is violating the patient's autonomy? Surely, he must tell the patient very strongly to modify his sexual behaviour. The doctor with a strict moral code could be forgiven for pointing out that "old-fashioned morals" are not so old-fashioned after all.

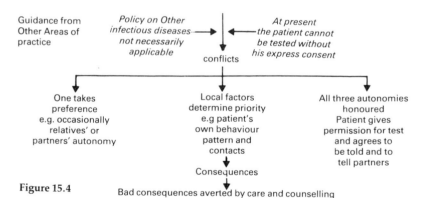

Figure 15.4

Screening

There are two aspects of this: first, it is very difficult to contain an epidemic when the authorities have no real idea of the size of the problem — the prevalence of the disease. It is important to find this out. Can it be done without breaking autonomy and confidentiality? Certainly by testing people and storing the data anonymously, as for any other disease, autonomy can be protected. The age and sex of the patient is important for plotting the distribution of the disease, but the individual name and address is not. Information of this sort is gleaned from blood given at blood transfusion centres, but blood donors do not necessarily present a random sample of the population. 'Local' factors may be important here in that insurance companies are starting to demand testing for HIV before issuing policies. In November 1988 the Minister of Health stated that there would be widespread *anonymous* testing of blood samples in order to establish the prevalence of the disease.

The second aspect of screening concerns the risk to doctors and nurses in caring for patients with undiagnosed HIV infection. Surgeons are particularly at risk through contact with infected blood. If they know a patient is HIV-positive they can take certain precautions to minimize the risk to all the theatre staff: this is standard practice with hepatitis-B-positive patients. But these precautions are expensive, adding about £100 to the cost of each operation and prolonging the operating time considerably. Here we have a direct conflict in the autonomy of the patient, who, under present guidelines, cannot be tested before operation without his expressed permission, and the autonomy of the surgeon and staff whose lives will be put at risk. It must clearly be understood that it is unethical for a doctor to refuse to treat an AIDS sufferer because he does not approve of his lifestyle (*see* Discussion and Ethical Codes p. 94), but doctors do have the autonomy to refuse to treat a patient under circumstances laid down by him (e.g., Jehovah's Witnesses). Surgeons *are* willing to treat the patient but are asking to be allowed to know what condition they are treating. The importance of knowing if the patient is carrying HIV has recently been highlighted by the suggestion that antiviral drugs may be effective if given as soon as a surgeon or nurse has been infected by a needle injury. This conflict is resolved at present in favour of the patient's autonomy but local factors again are likely to decide the issue. If surgeons are forced to treat all patients as if they have AIDS, the hospital service will grind to a standstill economically and in terms of the number of operations that can be done. This brings in the third aspect of autonomy — the rights of other patients who are waiting for treatment.

Isolation

This way of containing the disease has not been proposed but has certainly been discussed. Certainly, some countries are limiting the freedom of people to visit them without a negative HIV test. Should the HIV-positive person have the freedom, however, to spread the disease to others and so violate *their* freedom? The principle has been accepted in the past for other diseases, such as smallpox, but diseases are different in the way they are spread. Smallpox could easily be spread by casual contact, whereas, as far as we know at present, HIV infection is usually spread by sexual intercourse or the sharing of contaminated needles. Therefore, a positive decision has to be made by someone in order to contract the disease. He has the freedom *not* to catch it. Should people then be protected from themselves, a principle accepted in many safety regulations and in seat-belt legislation?

Education and exhortation and the provision of free needles to drug addicts have all been tried. Geographical isolation — so that the patient cannot spread the disease — would be a restriction of freedom on a scale unprecedented in peacetime, and would give governments enormous powers. In a country with very few sufferers it could be effective and might be justified; in some African countries, with such a huge prevalence of the disease, some segregation might be needed in the future for the small uninfected minority. These problems are real and urgent and governments have to grapple with them.

Summary

So where does our algorithm lead us?

From the decisions I have taken, I have reached the following conclusions. To:

1. Tell the truth to the patient and if he refuses to tell his spouse or partner, perhaps tell them if they are at real risk or, ideally, see them both together.

2. Agree to treat people who are HIV-positive but insist on preoperative screening so as not to violate the autonomy of the staff.

3. Use all methods of persuasion to stop the spread of the disease (short of isolation), and to tell uninfected people how to avoid being infected, as widespread government publicity has already done.

Some readers may have taken a different turn on one of the paths and ended up with different conclusions. For example, you may have decided that the patient's autonomy should take priority and that preoperative screening is not justified. Some might even have concluded that the risk to the population is so great that some form of isolation should be introduced. Others might put confidentiality as a top priority and not tell the sexual partner if the patient so wishes. In so doing, would you adopt the same policy with other, treatable, causes of sexually transmitted disease?

References and Further Reading

An Annotated Bibliography on Ethics and AIDS (1988). Bulletin no. 41.
  Institute of Medical Ethics.
AIDS—Medico-legal Advice (1988). Medical Defence Union.
Editorial (1990). Anonymous HIV testing. *Lancet*; **335**: 575–6.
General Medical Council (1988). *HIV Infection and AIDS: The Ethical
  Considerations.*

16 Animal research: cruelty or cure?

Research involving animals is the arena for a vigorous and important debate. On the one hand, there have been spectacular advances in treatment partly due to animal research — not least in the cure and care of cancer — on the other hand, animal right's movements have been increasingly vocal, and sometimes violent. Can this conflict be resolved? Who is right? Let us use our algorithm to dissect and analyse the problem.

Is there an ethical issue?

As mentioned in Chapter 4, this is a subject in which ethical and emotional issues are intertwined and confused. Research on animals, normally used as pets, provokes far more emotional reaction than research on frogs and snakes. But objections to animal research are not all emotional and many animal liberation workers passionately believe that such research involves important ethical principles: the exploitation of creatures that cannot give consent, is an abuse of man's power and demeans his status.

Which ethical components are involved?

Clearly the components are *aims, value* and, to a slight extent, *autonomy*. The central issue is the aim of the research, and there is a difference in degree, if not in kind, between research which aims to relieve childhood leukaemia and that which aims to check that the forty-fifth brand of hair shampoo to go on the market, does not damage the eyes. A number of people would make a firm distinction between research for therapeutic reasons and research for cosmetic reasons. In other words, to justify possible suffering to animals, there must be a worthy and important aim which takes precedence over suffering. Cosmetic research being a lower aim must produce minimum suffering. The relative value of animals in the scheme of things has already been mentioned in Chapter 7. Different religions and philosophers have widely differing views on the use of animals, not only for research, but also for food. Strict vegetarians who believe it is wrong to kill animals for food will consider it even more wrong to experiment on them. Buddhists have a profound respect for all life, however simple. On the other hand, some people with an entirely materialistic view of life might have no qualms about using animals in any way, provided it benefited themselves.

The question of *autonomy* is sometimes raised by animal rights groups and their argument goes like this: the main reason why animals should *not* be used is that they are unable to give consent, they have no autonomy, whereas humans are in a position to say 'No'. Therefore, these people would not oppose research on willing volunteers. This view was given publicity a few years ago in the debate over experiments with beagle dogs, who were made to smoke cigarettes so that manufacturers could produce a safer tobacco. A prominent public figure offered her services in place of the dogs! A similar argument can be applied to the difference between boxing, which is legal in Britain and dog fighting and cock fighting which is not. Boxers go into the ring voluntarily but animals do not. The very term 'animal rights' implies the defence of an autonomy which animals cannot possess unless humans give it to them. Therefore, so far, the algorithm looks like this:

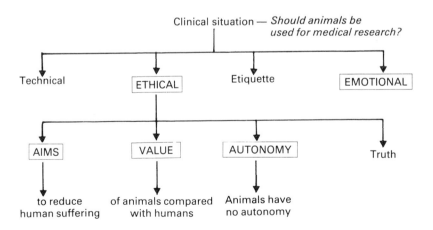

Figure 16.1

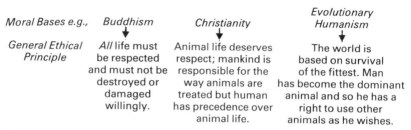

Figure 16.2

In Britain the consensus view is derived from Christian and some humanist views that animal research is justified but that respect for animals and animal suffering should always be a powerful consideration. This is the *specific ethical statement* that governs official animal research in Britain. But it is fair to say that this is not so in many countries round the world, even some 'highly developed' ones.

Ethical codes and the Law

There is no generally agreed ethical code governing animal research, as there is governing research with humans (Declaration of Helsinki, p. 97). There is also no compulsory animal ethical committee to review research projects, although referees and grant-giving bodies (and, indeed, editors of scientific journals) may well comment on the ethics of the animal work. In Britain, there is, however, legislation that goes back to 1876, which gives considerable power to the Home Office inspectors to check on animal research and to stop it if there is unnecessary suffering. All animal research workers have to be given a licence which approves

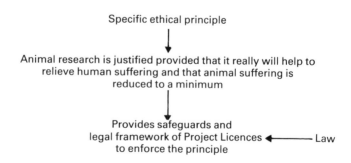

Figure 16.3

both the aims and methods of the research. This is first checked by a senior member of the scientific staff of the institution.

New legislation was adopted in 1986 (Animals—Scientific Procedures Act) and legislation will eventually be unified throughout the European Community. So here is an example where law fulfils a major function and has done for over 100 years. As with all laws, its effectiveness depends on those who administer it, but over the years, in general, inspectors have been very conscientious and animal research in Britain has not been abused, as it has in many countries. Some of the more extreme animal rights groups have taken examples from other countries, and used them in their campaigns, implying, if not stating, that these horrors were committed in Britain.

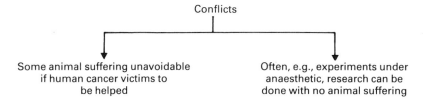

Figure 16.4

So we finish our algorithm by showing that with the conflicting values of man vs animals and human rights vs animal rights, the typical British compromise is to honour both by careful design of research, relief of animal suffering by analgesics and tight legal control. In other countries there is either absolute prohibition or a free-for-all.

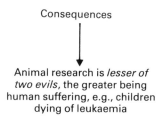

Figure 16.5

Consistency

Ethical consistency is important and it is so easy to apply our principles selectively. This puts those who do not accept any animal research in a difficult position. So many of the main medical advances have been due to animal research that it is dishonest to enjoy the benefits while condemning the methods. It must be very difficult to be a diabetic animal rights campaigner, because he is being kept alive by the results of the very research that he condemns. This brings in the fourth ethical component — integrity.

The future

This is not to say that scientists and animal groups alike should not work toward other methods of research, such as cell culture techniques. Because a particular method of research is 'allowable' or 'justifiable' it does not mean it is ideal. But at the present time there is no alternative to living animals for many areas of research, and it is important to safeguard and protect animals as much as possible. Some institutes have set up animal ethical research committees which check programmes before they are submitted for legal approval by the licensing body. This is a good development and will go some way to allaying the public's fear that many things may go on without the authority's knowledge.

Animal farm?

A new development involving animals is research on transplantation of animal organs such as pig kidneys into man. Some scientists are trying to make the organs compatible by introducing human genetic material into the pig so that it is incorporated into the growing kidney. The plan is then that this kidney will be recognized by the human immune system as being 'human'. Carried to its logical conclusion, each person could have a pet pig carrying spare parts for him! This research introduces a new ethical issue — the uniqueness and importance of human DNA — and brings into sharp focus the value of man and his relationship to animals. If 'a pig is but a horizontal human', as stated recently on television by a London transplant surgeon, then there is little problem. But if man is uniquely different from a pig, does this uniqueness lie in his genes or his spirit? Is there a fundamental difference between mixing genetic material and incorporating a pig's protein into our bodies when we eat bacon? Is this genetics research the 'slippery slope' leading to human/animal hybrids? As I write, the debate is just starting in the Sunday papers but it is likely to be very important.

References and Further Reading

Discussion on animal research has been characterised by polarisation of views and much emotion.

The Bulletin no. 46, published by the Institute of Medical Ethics (1989) has a report giving a summary of views and a lot of questions that need to be considered in justifying a piece of fundamental research.

Licensing details for animal work in Britain are obtained from the Home Office.

World Medical Association (1988) *Statement on Animal Use in Biomedical Research* quoted in Bulletin; **55:** 9–10 (1990) Institute of Medical Ethics.

17 Should healthcare staff take strike action?

This question has arisen in those countries whose medicine is State-controlled and where doctors and health workers are salaried by a monopoly employer — the Department of Health. It is unlikely to arise where there is fee-for-service payment or when doctors are self-employed. There is little difference, in the terms of employment, between a nurse with the British National Health Service and a factory worker in a large nationalised industry. Strike action has been taken in recent years in Britain by junior hospital doctors and many other hospital workers. Doctors have also taken strike action in other European countries and in Australia. The 'action' takes different forms but always involves refusal to see and treat certain groups of patients.

Is there an Ethical Question?

It might be argued that this is a matter of politics not ethics. But politics should have its ethics (as pointed out in Chapter 1) and

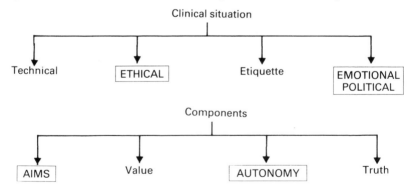

Figure 17.1

medical ethics *is* involved because the action concerns the right and wrong behaviour of health workers and it has an effect on the comfort, wellbeing and, sometimes, the safety of patients.

What are the ethical components?

The two components are the *aims* of medical care and its motivation, on the one hand, and *autonomy* of both health worker and patient, on the other. The question of strikes reveals, more than any other, people's underlying motives. People go on strike because they are dissatisfied with the pay or conditions of their job, or sometimes, because some right or privilege has been taken away or recognition not given, and sometimes in support of a colleague who they think has been wrongly treated. Strike action is only effective if the great majority take part, and someone, preferably the employer, is inconvenienced, embarrassed or harmed. It cannot be denied that throughout the world, making-money is one of the main motivations of most doctors. Even in countries like Britain, with its strong tradition of putting the patient first, the choice of specialties and work place is governed by consideration of comfort and pay.

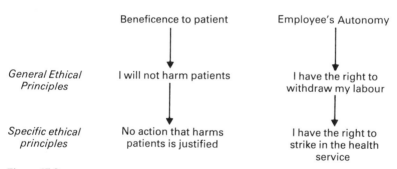

Figure 17.2

Aims

Only a few doctors put the challenge of the care of difficult and needy patients as their first priority. In countries such as the USA where huge sums can be made by doctors, the money motive becomes very strong and the popular specialties are those involving procedures, for which large fees can be charged: surgery, cardiology, endoscopy and now radiology. Because most health care is provided by private enterprise, the question of strike does not usually arise. Medicine is a profitable business. It would be interesting to guess how many doctors worldwide would still be in medicine if it was a relatively low status, low paid job — like nursing!

Autonomy

Autonomy first concerns the health workers. Most people would agree that, like other workers, they have the right to withdraw their labour. But if they exercise that right they may take away the rights of others — in this case the rights of patients to receive treatment. In a country with socialized medicine, neither the doctor nor the patient can turn to alternative sources for employment or medical care.

General and specific ethical principles

There are a number of ethical principles which are agreed by people with different moral backgrounds. The differences in the decision-making depend on the relative weighting given to each, and on the ultimate motivation. The following four specific principles arise from the general principle of caring for patients' needs, and the rights of employees:

1. The obligation to care for sick patients who cannot help themselves
2. The right of patients to expect such care from an organization which has offered or promised it
3. The right of workers to receive a 'fair' reward for their labour
4. The right of workers to withdraw their labour from the employer.

The great problem with the last principle is that it is impossible in a system, such as the British National Health Service to 'hurt' the employer without harming the patient — in fact, it is difficult to harm the employer at all, except in terms of reduced votes at the next general election. The following spurious argument was used by some junior doctors to justify strike action: a strike, although harming patients in the short term will be to their benefit in the long term, because a well-paid doctor is a happy doctor and he will treat them much better in the future!

The place of law

The law in Britain now has specific limits about the right to strike and the way a decision to strike is made. This has changed since the strike which brought hospitals to a standstill, only a few years ago.

The ethical codes

These are specific on the duty to patients. The Declaration of Geneva (p. 94) states: "The health of my patient will be my first consideration' and would seem to outlaw strikes for personal gain. The statement 'I will not permit consideration of religion, nationality . . . party politics . . . to intervene between my duty and my patients' obviously outlaws withdrawal of care from the patient for political ends.

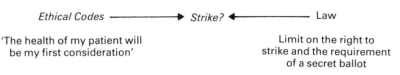

Figure 17.3

Conflicting principles

There is a direct conflict between the needs of the patient and the rights and autonomy of the doctor (or other health worker). If withdrawing labour does *not* harm patients in some way, then the value of the job should be questioned! However, some posts obviously have more direct effect on patients than others. When there have been strikes in the NHS, the striking groups have actually continued to treat life-threatening emergencies. But it is those patients waiting for semiurgent or non-urgent treatment, often for painful conditions, that have suffered. How can this conflict be resolved?

Some groups, like the Royal College of Nursing, have adopted a 'through-way' policy and stated clearly that they will not strike and that their overriding duty is to the patient. They have used other methods of persuasion and have rallied public support, but have stopped short of strike action.

Other groups, e.g., the junior hospital doctors and some health service unions have taken strike action and tried to minimize harm to very ill patients. In the past, some militant union officials have ignored patients' needs and turned off the heating to young children's wards or tried to prevent oxygen cylinders coming into a hospital. They have put *their* rights clearly above those of the patients, who of course are in no position to exert theirs. In these cases, hospitals and patients have been used as pawns in an ideological conflict.

Yet other groups have taken a middle road and let 'local factors' determine priority by taking very specific and limited, short-term action which has been carefully planned.

Possibly the only way of honouring *both* conflicting principles is to resign from the health service, thereby asserting one's right on autonomy — and then treating the patients on a freelance basis. This

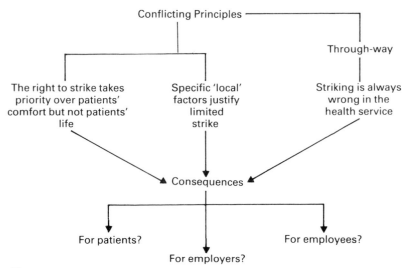

Figure 17.4

is possible for some doctors, but difficult for other groups of workers in the hospital service and could have disastrous results for future careers unless it was done by all the staff at once, who then offered their services back to the hospital, at a particular fee.

The other situation when strike action or withdrawal of labour might be justified is if the employer asked an employee to do something that was against his conscience. To take a far-fetched example: if the employer insisted that all patients who had been in the hospital for more than three months, and were over 80 years old, should be sent home or be given a large dose of morphine, because they were 'blocking beds', this might well conflict with people's ethical principles and justify 'strike' action against the employer.

However, it is to be hoped that this situation will not arise again; and that the important principle, of caring for others' needs, will enable employers and the better-paid staff to be aware of the conditions of lower-paid employees, and do something about it before serious problems arise. It would also seem reasonable for a 'no strike' clause to be in the contract of those who undertake the responsible job of caring for the sick.

References and Further Reading

Drookin G (1977). Strikes and the National Health Service: some legal and ethical issues. *Journal of Medical Ethics*; **3**: 76–82.

Royal College of Nursing (1977). Code of professional conduct: a discussion document. *Journal of Medical Ethics*; **3**: 115–23.

18 Fetal brain cell transplants — hope or horror?

A new ethical problem has resulted from recent attempts to transplant fetal brain cells into patients with Parkinsonism. The scientific basis for this work is that fetal brain cells are rich in dopamine, which is lacking in part of the brain of these patients, and fetal cells are not rejected by the recipient in the same way as adult donor tissues. Parkinson's disease is a distressing condition, affecting thousands of people, who at present have to take drugs continuously, often with only partial relief. We will now examine this problem which to some people seems a wonderful new advance, but to others, science horror fiction becoming a reality.

Is there an ethical problem?

There certainly is! But even here, there is a significant emotional element and, possibly, as we will see, a technical question as well. In the same way that early heart transplants caused anxiety, because the heart was considered the seat of the emotions, any talk of 'brain' transplants conjures up visions of transferring thoughts or 'personality'. So it is important to be clear that, at the present time, there is no plan to transplant 'brains' to produce supermen or Frankenstein monsters, but merely to inject a few isolated cells which will stay alive and produce a missing chemical.

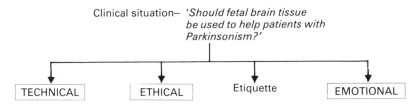

Clinical situation— *'Should fetal brain tissue be used to help patients with Parkinsonism?'*

TECHNICAL   ETHICAL   Etiquette   EMOTIONAL

Figure 18.1

What are the ethical components?

Most countries and most philosophies (except, for example, Jehovah's Witnesses) have come to accept that whole organ transplants of kidneys or livers are ethical. However there were three early stumbling blocks.

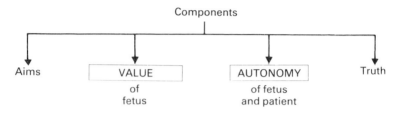

Figure 18.2

The main problem was of *autonomy* for both the donor and the recipient. Some thought that the personal uniqueness of an individual was being violated by his receiving another person's organ (but the same people happily accepted blood transfusion). The second aspect of autonomy was the difficulty obtaining consent from the donor's relatives and giving them legal authority on behalf of the brain-dead patient. The third issue turned out to be technical rather than ethical: how to determine that the donor was indeed brain-dead. No one was suggesting, seriously, that brain-damaged patients should be 'killed' to obtain their organs for transplantation (despite some scare-mongering by the media at the time). The difficulty was to be sure that the donor was brain-dead, before removing his kidneys. Therefore, a series of criteria and safeguards was devised which were accepted nationally and internationally (Declaration of Sydney, p. 95). Organ transplantation has been a field where there has been a remarkable degree of ethical agreement, but there is still profound public fear that donors may not be 'brain dead'; this was well-illustrated by the 'exposure' on television of unsubstantiated reports of patients, who had recovered, but at some stage had fulfilled the criteria of brain death. This had a long and severe effect on the number of donors for transplantation; and the admission by the doctors concerned, that they had not checked the facts, did not reverse the trend.

How then does fetal brain transplant differ from the well-established practice of renal transplantation? The answer is in the nature of the donor and its value and autonomy.

Moral basis and general ethical principles

The same issues arise here as with abortion in general. If the value and status of the fetus is no different from the value of the gallbladder or kidney, then the mother has the same right to donate

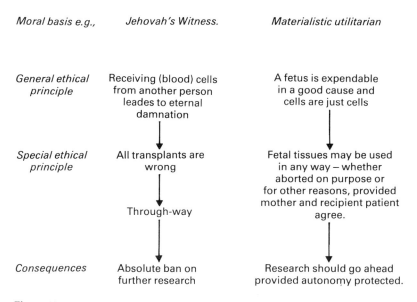

Moral basis e.g.,	*Jehovah's Witness.*	*Materialistic utilitarian*
General ethical principle	Receiving (blood) cells from another person leades to eternal damnation	A fetus is expendable in a good cause and cells are just cells
Special ethical principle	All transplants are wrong Through-way	Fetal tissues may be used in any way – whether aborted on purpose or for other reasons, provided mother and recipient patient agree.
Consequences	Absolute ban on further research	Research should go ahead provided autonomy protected.

Figure 18.3

her fetus to help someone else, as she has to donate her kidney to a relative in need. If the fetus, by contrast, is regarded as being as valuable as a fully grown human being, then, if the fetus dies or is aborted spontaneously, there is an exact parallel with transplantation from a brain-dead donor. This then becomes a technical challenge: is it possible to retrieve viable brain cells from a spontaneous abortion? In between, is the possibility of retrieving fetuses from truly therapeutic abortions, and then growing the brain cells in tissue culture to produce a line of cells, which can be used for a number of patients.

Therefore, the ethical issue is the same as that in the early days of kidney transplantation — how is the donor organ obtained?

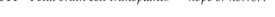

To provide safeguards and controls ⟵———————— Law
and to respect conscientious objection

Figure 18.4

Conflict of principles and possible consequences

One can foresee the conflict between the needs of the patient with Parkinsonism and an unhappily pregnant relative! There may even be pressure on people to become pregnant specially to provide donor cells. The conflict is between the desire to do good to one patient (beneficence) and the value and autonomy of a fetus.

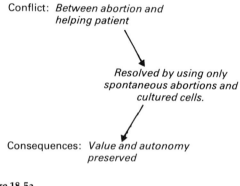

Conflict: *Between abortion and helping patient*

Resolved by using only spontaneous abortions and cultured cells.

Consequences: *Value and autonomy preserved*

Figure 18.5a

Consequences

Slippery slope?

Figure 18.5b

Consistency

This issue illustrates well the importance of consistency with other transplant practice and a parallel with other areas. Established transplant practice would reject the production of fetuses or their termination especially for donor purposes. On the other hand, some attitudes to the fetus would tend to promote this practice.

As with *in vitro* fertilization, technical improvement may well simplify the ethical dilemma, but at this stage safeguards must be established quickly to prevent exploitation of fetuses. The Warnock

Committee provided guidelines which could well be extended to cover this problem and provide a basis of law. But even within a legal framework, there are bound to be variations in practice, depending on individual moral views, and some will be very unhappy in accepting the 'benefits' resulting from therapeutic abortion.

References and Further Reading

Gillon R (1988). Ethics of fetal brain cell transplants. *British Medical Journal*; **296**: 1212–3.

Jones DG (1987). *Manufacturing Humans*. Inter-Varsity Press, Leicester.

Review (1989). *Evidence to the Polkinghorne Committee: what should one be allowed to do to a fetus?* Bulletin no. 49. Institute of Medical Ethics.

Review of the Guidance on the Research Use of Fetuses and Fetal Material 1989 ("The Polkinghorne Report") KM762 HMSO.

World Medical Association (1989). Statement on Fetal Tissue Transplantation, quoted in *Bulletin of Medical Ethics* (1990); **55**: 80.

19 Voluntary euthanasia: crime or kindness?

Euthanasia is never out of the limelight for long. Many of the arguments have been mentioned already in this book but will be brought together and summarized here.

Is there an ethical question?

The problem with the euthanasia debate is not any doubt about its ethical importance, but confusion over its varied definitions. The different meanings have been given on p. 83, but for there to be any meaningful debate, we must confine our definition to the intentional immediate ending of a patient's life ('suicide by proxy') by a doctor or nurse, at the request of the patient or his designated

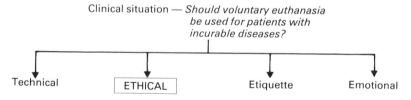

Clinical situation — *Should voluntary euthanasia be used for patients with incurable diseases?*

Technical   ETHICAL   Etiquette   Emotional

Figure 19.1

relative. Compulsory euthanasia, of the handicapped, for example, is not being contemplated at the present time but, as we shall see, the law would not be a very good safeguard.

What are the ethical components?

The two components are *aim* and *autonomy*. One of the fundamental aims of medical care is 'beneficence', whereas killing a patient can hardly be construed as 'doing no harm'. But on the other hand, relief of suffering and pain *is* the aim of care, and relieving pain by putting

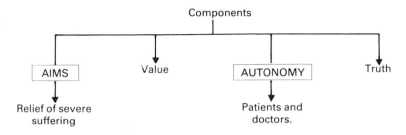

Figure 19.2

an end to the patient's misery could be considered beneficent. The second component — *autonomy* — affects doctors, patients and relatives. As we have seen, when analysing the Karen Quinlan case (p. 109–110) a patient has the right to refuse treatment: does this autonomy extend to asking for euthanasia? As with the debate on abortion, the doctor's (or nurse's) autonomy must also be preserved — they must not be forced to do something against their principles and consciences.

Moral basis and general ethical principles

This question brings into sharp relief the fundamental difference between a theistic and atheist view of the universe, and of human personality and responsibility.

The humanist is the 'master of his fate and the captain of his soul' because he does not believe in a God to whom he is answerable. A God-fearing person believes he is answerable to God for the way he

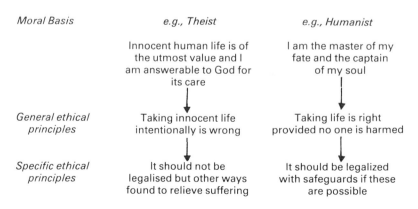

Figure 19.3

spends and ends his life (if this is within his control). Most people have relatives and dependents to whom they are either a support or a burden, and their rights need to be considered.

So the general ethical principle for the theistic would be that the intentional taking of innocent life is wrong and they should look to other means of controlling pain and suffering (which they have demonstrated through the hospice movement). Some would have the extreme view that anything that even shortens life is wrong. For the atheist, the ethical principle is that he has the right to take his own life, provided it does not harm or distress other people.

The place of law and ethical codes

All the ethical codes reject euthanasia explicity or implicity. The law in Britain forbids it (see discussion in Chapter 13). There have

Codes ⟶ Both forbid active euthanasia implicitly or explicitly ⟵ Law

Figure 19.4

been a number of attempts to alter the law, the most recent being in the form of an amendment to the Suicide Bill by making it no longer a crime to *assist* someone's suicide, as it is no longer a crime to attempt suicide. As quoted on p. 105, some of those concerned with trying to draft the Euthanasia Bill have realized how difficult it is to provide safeguards. Unfortunately, the Dr Arthur trial (p. 110) failed to clarify the situation and provide legal guidance for the borderline case. One of the bills put before Parliament some years ago referred to 'painful, incurable disease' as grounds for euthanasia; but this would cover most forms of arthritis and illustrates the difficulty of wording a meaningful law. However, any law must safeguard the doctor's conscience; indeed, if a law should be passed, the best solution might be to set up 'euthanasia centres', with trained technicians and advisory lawyers, and divorce it completely from normal medical care.

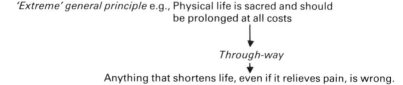

'Extreme' general principle e.g., Physical life is sacred and should be prolonged at all costs

Through-way

Anything that shortens life, even if it relieves pain, is wrong.

Figure 19.5

Conflicting ethical principles

The humanist does not have any real conflict, provided certain safeguards are met. But the theist has this conflict: between not killing on the one hand but relieving suffering on the other. He can resolve this conflict by using other means of relieving pain and researching into newer and better methods. If the pain relief does

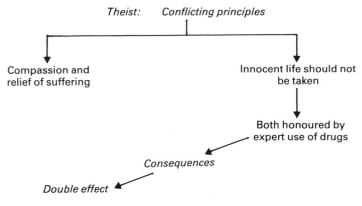

Figure 19.6

shorten life, which it usually does *not*, then he takes refuge in the principle of double effect. If the symptoms cannot be completely relieved despite full dose of drug, he will still give priority to preservation of life, or rather, not 'killing' intentionally.

The slippery slope

One of the anxieties about any euthanasia law is that it is the start of the slippery slope — that voluntary euthanasia under extreme circumstances will become euthanasia on request (as has happened with abortion, after the 1967 Act). The ever greater anxiety is that voluntary euthanasia will imperceptibly change to compulsory euthanasia for the handicapped and elderly.

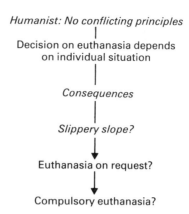

Humanist: No conflicting principles

Decision on euthanasia depends
on individual situation

Consequences

Slippery slope?

Euthanasia on request?

Compulsory euthanasia?

Figure 19.7

References and Further Reading

Three books, written around the time of Lord Raglan's Bill, gave views from many different philosophical standpoints and illustrate the background to the debate.

Downing AV (ed) (1969). *Euthanasia and the Right to Death.* Peter Owen, London.

Gould J and Craigmyle Lord (1971). *Your Death Warrant?* Geoffrey Chapman, London.

Vere D (1971). *Voluntary Euthanasia — Is There an Alternative?* Christian Medical Fellowship, London.

Brahams D (1990) Euthanasia in the Netherlands. *Lancet;* **335:** 591–2.

British Medical Association (1988). Euthanasia: conclusions of a BMA working party. *British Medical Journal;* **296:,** 1376–7.

Institute of Medical Ethics (1988). *A Review of Euthanasia and Living Wills* (Bulletin 38).

20 Choices

Throughout this book the emphasis has been on the need and duty to take decisions. There are many choices to make in the practice of medicine and many of them have ethical implications. However, the one choice we are not free to make is to opt out of ethics and still practice medicine! The ethics and the practice of medicine are inextricably bound together and you will still be making ethical decisions even if you decide to have nothing to do with the study of ethics. Not everybody needs to study medical ethics in great detail or as an elective subject, but all need to be aware of its framework and principles.

The most important choice by far is the choice of a world view — the moral base that will govern your practice of medicine. We have seen in Chapter 5 that there are a number of very different world views that, if they are allowed to influence decisions, will lead to very different results. Perhaps you would prefer to pick and choose using one moral code in one situation and a different one for another situation: unfortunately that is not really allowed! If you do that, then your ethics becomes *situational* which, as Ian Kennedy (1982) points out, is not really ethics at all. The choice of a moral basis is made on whether you think it is true, consistent and that it leads to decisions and actions which you consider are the most valuable — in other words, whether it works. But even with the best ethical basis and logical system of thought, we still sometimes find confusion and our way is obstructed at the end of the path. The ethical jungle, rather than clearing, closes in around us and our nice broad path peters out into a group of tiny winding tracks that appear to lead nowhere (Fig. 20.1). *Some ethical problems are never solved.*

Why do ethics not always work?

There are at least three main reasons:
- False expectations
- Human nature
- Lack of Motivation

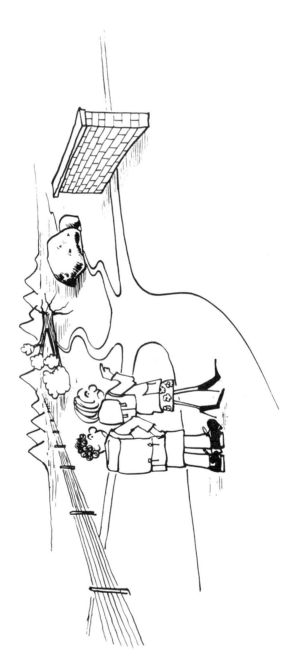

Figure 20.1 Some ethical problems are never *solved* — the paths merely peter out

False expectations

These are mentioned at the beginning in Chapter 1. Many people have a false expectation of what ethical reasoning can achieve. We demand *resolution* or *solution* of problems rather in the same way as we demand solution of a crossword puzzle or a chess problem. But in some dilemmas in medicine, there will be *no* solution, in that sense. We may have to hold two opposing principles in tension. We are practising medicine in a non-ideal world, and trying to apply ideals to medical practice is not different from applying them to other walks of life. The fact that we cannot always resolve a problem does not mean that we should immediately abandon the ideals. It means we will often have to take difficult decisions and will have to feel some of the unresolved tension that these decisions involve. It means that we sometimes have to be satisfied with a compromise solution and make the best decision under the circumstances from the evidence available, knowing that we may be wrong. As in other walks of life, we must learn from our mistakes. The Pond Report also encouraged students 'to make, defend, criticise and reflect on the kind of moral judgements which medical practice will require of them'. It is perfectly correct for a student to argue the case of his or her view and to analyse where each leads. The student should take the time to do this before his decisions directly affect patients. Sometimes two people start from the same moral basis and end up with a different decision in practice. Others starting from two quite different moral viewpoints find themselves agreeing on a line of action. We must also respect those with a different viewpoint, genuinely held, even if we cannot agree with them.

> The ultimate purpose (of ethics) is to construct and defend a coherent moral theory for medical practice based on current principles applying to all . . . this 'Holy Grail' has certainly not been reached and may well be essentially unobtainable.
>
> Gillon, 1986

The problem of human nature

The second problem lies in doctors and patients themselves rather than the rules and principles they construct — that is in human nature itself. Throughout history, some people all of the time, and everybody some of the time, have failed to keep even man-made rules for the smooth running of society. Everyone has a tendency to be selfish on occasions and to be influenced by status, money, popularity and appearances and to manipulate others for his own purpose. Human beings also tend to be inconsistent, behaving in one way in one situation and very differently in another. Consistency is often discussed in relationship to the following question: 'Does it matter how someone behaves in private so long as his or her public or professional life is ethical?' or more specifically 'Should a doctor be disciplined by the profession for moral lapses which do not involve his patients or any of his professional relationships?' The problem of answering 'No' to these questions is the assumption that different aspects of life can be kept in two water-tight compartments — that a doctor can steal in his spare time but not steal from his patients. If for no other reason than patient confidence, a doctor's moral behaviour has to be higher than the average member of society at large. If doctors and nurses stole, as many people steal, a patient would not dare to take his jacket off in the surgery or the outpatient clinic! Why should a person who is quite undisciplined and uncontrolled in private dealings, suddenly change when operating or dealing with patients? For these reasons, the public and the profession have to be concerned about other aspects of a doctor's behaviour than that shown purely at work, and the General Medical Council may take note of court cases involving doctor's misdemeanours such as drunken driving or financial embezzlement. The assumption that the doctor's ethical standards are high gives them the right, for example, to countersign passport application forms in the same way as a minister of religion or a solicitor. The important question is: 'Where does a person get the power to do what he knows to be right?' Is he capable of changing himself and his society by his own efforts or does he need to transcend his environment and have a reference point outside himself. Medical ethics have no answer to these problems of human nature, apart from its disciplinary machinery and, ultimately, the rule of law. But some of the faiths that give rise to ethical principles also say quite a bit about the moral failure of human beings and its solution (*see* pp. 40–42).

Motivation

Allied to the problem of moral weakness and failure, is the problem of motivation. Ethical guidelines and codes are doomed to fail unless the majority of doctors and healthcare workers want to practise in an ethical way and *wish* to put the patient's interests above money-making and any other selfish motives. Lord Lister, the father of antiseptic surgery, was fond of saying that 'The one rule of practice is to put yourself in the patient's place' — a medical paraphrase of the well known biblical injunction to 'Do to others what you would have them to do to you'. That is a fine ideal, but where does this motivation, this compassion come from? Why should we be concerned about another suffering human being when his suffering has no direct bearing on us? Again, we must go back to basic insights and revelations: man's capacity for *altruistic* love must come from outside himself; it is not 'natural'.

Some ethicists argue that motivation is the most important factor. If motivation is right, all else falls into place and if motivation is wrong, nothing else will work. They propose an ethic of 'virtue' rather than ethic of principles and rules. Good people, they say, will act in a good way and therefore our efforts should be directed towards changing people rather than elaborating ethical codes. Much of this is true and, therefore, motivation does matter enormously. Aristotle, Hume and Augustine from different backgrounds, all insisted that the will, rather than the reason alone, is the decisive factor in moral decisions. But there are two snags:

1. 'Mankind has an almost limitless ability to convince himself that what he wants to do is morally justifiable' (Smithalls, 1973, q.v.). Without some checks and standards, motivation alone can be deceptive.
2. Any action will be justified by being done 'from the best of motives'. The aims will justify the means in true Machiavellian style.

For these reasons, motives alone are not enough. Motives and ethical principles must go together in the same way that its engine powers a car along a certain road.

In ethical matters, wisdom is required more than knowledge and wisdom is in short supply. While the teleologist looks for more knowledge to solve the problem of dangerous knowledge, the deontologist echoes the old Jewish proverb 'The fear of the Lord is the beginning of wisdom'. Sometimes those who question the ethics of new medical advances are regarded as reactionary and out of touch with modern thinking: ethical decisions often take considerable courage.

In Britain, and in many other parts of the world, the ethical practice of medicine has relied on the altruistic and voluntary acceptance of agreed standards by the great majority of the profession. In places, this altruism and dedication are growing rather cool. It is the purpose of this book to question and re-kindle motives and to encourage a new generation of students to think clearly and courageously on ethical matters, so that the tremendous advances in medical technology may be controlled and directed to the true wellbeing of all.

References and Further Reading

Gillon R (1986). *Philosophical Medical Ethics*. John Wiley, Chichester.
Kennedy IM (1982). Rethinking medical ethics. *Journal of the Royal College of Surgeons of Edinburgh;* **22**: 1–8.
Smithalls RW and Beard RW (1973). New horizons in medical ethics: research investigations and the foetus. *British Medical Journal;* **2**: 464.

Appendix I

University of Sheffield: Annual Degree Congregations

Chancellor, I wish to remind the graduates and graduands about to be presented to you of the main tenets of the Hippocratic Oath that have guided our practice for more than 2000 years:

1. I will remain loyal to the high traditions and responsibilities of my profession
2. My patients' health and welfare will be my paramount consideration. I will do my best for my patients at all times and refrain from any action which may be harmful
3. I will, in the course of my work, come into special relationships with my fellow human beings calling for great propriety and trust. I will avoid all wrong-doing and anything mischievous or dishonourable
4. Whatsoever I see or hear during my practice that ought to be kept secret, I will not divulge.

Appendix II

Addresses of Profesional Organizations Referred to in Text

Institute of Medical Ethics
151 Great Portland Street, London W1N 5PB
Tel. 071–580–5282
(Bulletins are issued monthly)

The General Medical Council
44 Hallam Street, London W1N 6AE
Tel. 071–580–7642

United Kingdom Central Council for Nursing, Midwifery and
Health Visiting
23 Portland Place, London W1N 3AF
Tel. 071–637–7181

Council for Professions Supplementary to Medicine
Park House, 184 Kennington Park Road, London SE11 4BU
Tel. 071–582–0866

British Medical Association
BMA House, Tavistock Square, London WC1H 9JP
Tel. 071–387–4499

Royal College of Nursing
Henrietta Place, London W1M 0AV
Tel. 071–409–3333

British Association of Social Workers
16 Kent Street, Birmingham B5 6RD
Tel. 021–622–3911

British Association of Occupational Therapists
20 Rede Place, Off Chepstow Place, London W2 4TU
Tel. 071–229–9738/9

British Association of Physiotherapists
14 Bedford Row, London WC1R 4ED
Tel. 071–242–1941

The Royal College of Radiographers
14 Upper Wimpole Street, London W1M 8BN
Tel. 071–935–5726

Medical Defence Union
3 Devonshire Place, London W1N 2EA
Tel. 071–486–6181

Medical Protection Society
50 Hallam Street, London W1
Tel. 071–637–0541

Medical and Dental Defence Union of Scotland
144 West George Street, Glasgow G2 2HW
Tel. 041–332–6646

Royal College of Physicians of London
11 St. Andrews Place, London NW1 4LE
Tel. 071–935–1174

Christian Medical Fellowship
157 Waterloo Road, London SE1 8UU
Tel. 071–928–4694

USA

Northwest Institute of Ethics and the Life Sciences
72, 5th Avenue, New York, NY 1001

Publish *Bioethics Quarterly*

Institute of Society, Ethics and the Life Sciences
360 Broadway, Hastings on Hudson NY 10706

Publish *The Hastings Centre Reports*

American Medical Association
535 North Dearborn Street, Chicago, ILL 60610 4377
Tel. 0101 312 645 4818

Worldwide

World Health Organization (WHO)
Ave. Appla 1211, Geneva 27, Switzerland
Tel. 01091 21 11

World Medical Association
28 Ave. des Alpes, 01201 Ferney-Voltaire, France
Telex 385755

Appendix III

Further reading

Byrne, Peter (ed.) (1990). *Medicine, medical ethics and the value of life.* Wiley, 1990.

Byrne, Peter (ed.) (1986) *Rights and wrongs in medicine.* Oxford University Press.

Dowie, Jack (1988). *Professional judgement: reader in clinical decision making.* Cambridge University Press.

Elford R.J. (1987). *Medical ethics and elderly people.* Churchill Livingstone.

Fulford, K.W.M. (1989). *Moral theory and medical practice.* Cambridge University Press.

Humphrey, Derek *(et al)* (1986). *Right to die: understanding euthanasia.* Bodley Head.

Jacob, J. M. (1988). *Doctors and rules: a sociology of professional values.* Routledge.

Kuhse, Helga (1987). *Sanctity of life doctrine in medicine: a critique.* Oxford University Press.

Mason J.K. (1988). *Human life and medical practice.* Edinburgh University Press.

Mason, J.K. *(et al)* (1987). *Law and medical ethics.* 2nd ed. Butterworths.

Menzel, Paul T (1990). *Strong medicine: ethical rationing of health care.* Oxford University Press.

Rowley, Peter T. (ed.) (1989). *New medical genetics: probing social and ethical issues.* Oxford University Press.

Reiser, Stanley *(et al)* (eds) (1977). *Ethics in medicine.* MIT Press.

Kennedy, Ian (1987). *Treat me right.* Oxford University Press.

Hull, Richard T. (1989). *Ethical issues in the new reproductive technologies*. Wadsworth.

Rogers, John (1988). *Medical ethics, human choices*. Herald Press.

Dunstan, G. R. and Shinebourne, Elliot A. (1989). *Doctors' decisions*. Oxford University Press.

Index